POCKET GUIDE to
Addiction Assessment and Treatment

D0881774

POCKET GUIDE to
Addiction Assessment and Treatment

Edited by

Petros Levounis, M.D., M.A.

Erin Zerbo, M.D.

Rashi Aggarwal, M.D.

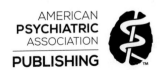

AMERICAN
PSYCHIATRIC
ASSOCIATION
PUBLISHING

Copyright © 2016 American Psychiatric Association
ALL RIGHTS RESERVED

Manufactured in the United States of America on acid-free paper
20   19   18   17   16   5   4   3   2   1
First Edition

Typeset in Palatino LT Std and Trade Gothic LT Std.

American Psychiatric Association Publishing
1000 Wilson Boulevard
Arlington, VA 22209-3901
www.appi.org

Library of Congress Cataloging-in-Publication Data
Names: Levounis, Petros, editor. | Zerbo, Erin, 1981– , editor. | Aggarwal, Rashi, 1973– , editor. | American Psychiatric Association.
Title: Pocket guide to addiction assessment and treatment / edited by Petros Levounis, Erin Zerbo, Rashi Aggarwal.
Description: First edition. | Arlington, VA : American Psychiatric Association Publishing, [2016] | Includes bibliographical references and index.
Identifiers: LCCN 2016007672 | ISBN 9781585625123 (alk. paper)
Subjects: | MESH: Substance-Related Disorders | Substance-Related Disorders—therapy | Handbooks
Classification: LCC RC564 | NLM WM 34 | DDC 616.86—dc23
LC record available at http://lccn.loc.gov/2016007672

British Library Cataloguing in Publication Data
A CIP record is available from the British Library.

Contents

PART I
Fundamentals of Addiction

1 **Neurobiology of Addiction**
From Reward to Relief: The Complex
Neuroadaptations Underlying Addiction

National Institute on Drug Abuse

2 **Addiction Assessment Across
Settings of Care**
Approaches for the Twenty-First Century

Mirela Feurdean, M.D.

3 **DSM-5 Diagnosis and Toxicology.**

Petros Levounis, M.D., M.A.
Lindsay Lynch, B.S.

PART II
Substances and Behaviors

4 **Alcohol**

Faye Chao, M.D.
Nauman Ashraf, M.D.

PART III
Treatment

Contributors

Rashi Aggarwal, M.D.
Associate Professor of Psychiatry, Rutgers New Jersey Medical School, Newark, New Jersey

Nauman Ashraf, M.D.
Medical Director, Inpatient Psychiatry Unit, Ozark Center; Interim Program Director, Osteopathic Psychiatry Residency Program, Ozark Center, Joplin, Missouri

Jonathan Avery, M.D.
Assistant Professor of Psychiatry, Weill Cornell Medical College, New York, New York

Tshering Bhutia, M.B.B.S.
Resident in Psychiatry, Rutgers New Jersey Medical School, Newark, New Jersey

Timothy Koehler Brennan, M.D., M.P.H.
Director, Fellowship in Addiction Medicine, The Addiction Institute of New York, New York

Faye Chao, M.D.
Assistant Professor of Psychiatry, Icahn School of Medicine at Mount Sinai, and Unit Chief of Inpatient Addiction Services, The Addiction Institute at Mount Sinai West Hospital, New York, New York

Adam R. Demner, M.D.
Assistant Clinical Professor of Psychiatry, New York University Langone Medical Center, New York, New York

Emily Deringer, M.D.
Clinical Assistant Professor of Psychiatry, New York University School of Medicine, New York, New York

John Douglas, M.D., M.B.A.
Clinical Director, Outpatient Addiction Program, Silver Hill Hospital, New Canaan, Connecticut

Mirela Feurdean, M.D.
Assistant Professor of Medicine, Rutgers New Jersey Medical School, Newark, New Jersey

Timothy Fong, M.D.
Professor of Psychiatry, Semel Institute for Neuroscience and Human Behavior at UCLA; Co-Director, UCLA Gambling Studies Program; Program Director, Addiction Psychiatry Fellowship, University of California, Los Angeles

Bernadine Han, M.D., M.S.
Psychiatry Resident, New York-Presbyterian Hospital/Payne Whitney Clinic, New York, New York

Shaojie Han, M.D., M.S.
Fellow in Addiction Psychiatry, Albert Einstein College of Medicine, Bronx, New York

Grace Hennessy, M.D.
Director, Substance Abuse Recovery Program, Department of Veterans Affairs, New York Harbor Health Care System, New York Campus; Clinical Assistant Professor of Psychiatry, New York University School of Medicine, New York, New York

Abigail J. Herron, D.O.
Director of Psychiatry, The Institute for Family Health; Assistant Professor of Psychiatry, Mt. Sinai School of Medicine, New York, New York

Vicki Kalira, M.D.
Clinical Assistant Professor of Psychiatry, New York University Langone Medical Center, New York

Cheryl A. Kennedy, M.D.
Associate Professor of Psychiatry, Rutgers New Jersey Medical School, Newark, New Jersey

Michael A. Ketteringham, M.D., M.P.H.
Medical Director of Consultation Psychiatry, Staten Island University Hospital, Staten Island, New York

Sonya Lazarevic, M.D., M.S.
Private practice, New York, New York

Annie Lévesque, M.D.
Fellow in Addiction Medicine, The Addiction Institute of New York, New York

Petros Levounis, M.D., M.A.
Chair, Department of Psychiatry, Rutgers New Jersey Medical School; Chief of Service, University Hospital, Newark, New Jersey

Lindsay Lynch, B.S.
Third-Year Medical Student, Rutgers New Jersey Medical School, Newark, New Jersey

Douglas Opler, M.D.
Assistant Professor of Psychiatry, Rutgers New Jersey Medical School, Newark, New Jersey

C. Alexander Paleos, M.D.
Clinical Assistant Professor of Psychiatry, New York University School of Medicine, New York, New York

Caylin Riley, B.S.
Kansas City University of Medicine and Biosciences, Kansas City, Missouri

Maryn Sloane, M.D.
Fellow in Addiction Psychiatry, Division of Alcoholism and Substance Abuse, New York University/Bellevue Hospital Center, New York; Director, Chemical Dependency Services, North American Partners in Pain Management, Second Chance Clinic, Long Island, New York

J. David Stiffler, M.D.
Clinical Assistant Professor of Psychiatry, New York University School of Medicine, New York

Alex Zaphiris, M.D., M.S.
Clinical Instructor, Department of Family and Community Medicine, University of California, San Francisco

Erin Zerbo, M.D.
Assistant Professor of Psychiatry, Rutgers New Jersey Medical School, Newark, New Jersey

Disclosures

The following contributors have declared all forms of support received within the 12 months before manuscript submission that may represent a competing interest in relation to their work published in this volume, as follows:

Timothy Fong, M.D.   *Speaker's Bureau:* Reckitt-Benckiser; *Research:* Bridges to Recovery

The following contributors have stated that they have no competing interests during the year preceding manuscript submission:

Nauman Ashraf, M.D.; Jonathan Avery, M.D.; Tshering Bhutia, M.B.B.S.; Timothy Koehler Brennan, M.D., M.P.H.; Faye Chao, M.D.; Adam R. Demner, M.D.; Emily Deringer, M.D.; John Douglas, M.D., M.B.A.; Mirela Feurdean, M.D.; Bernadine Han, M.D., M.S.; Shaojie Han, M.D., M.S.; Grace Hennessy, M.D.; Abigail J. Herron, D.O.; Vicki Kalira, M.D.; Cheryl A. Kennedy, M.D.; Sonya Lazarevic, M.D., M.S.; Annie Lévesque, M.D.; Petros Levounis, M.D., M.A.; Douglas Opler, M.D.; Caylin Riley, B.S.; Maryn Sloane, M.D.; J. David Stiffler, M.D.; Alex Zaphiris, M.D., M.S.; Erin Zerbo, M.D.

Preface

This is not a textbook.

It is not even a handbook or a manual. It's a pocket guide, a compact helper for the enthusiastic, yet not necessarily experienced, traveler in the world of addiction.

When we first thought about writing this book, we asked ourselves the following questions:

- What would I have liked to know about assessing and treating addiction when I first started?
- When textbooks feel overwhelming, the Internet is not consistently trustworthy, and helpful colleagues seem overextended, where do I turn?
- What information does a clinician need to have to optimally serve her or his patients in today's health care environment?

Patients with substance use disorders can be some of the most vexing and challenging patients, and practitioners often struggle with these patients' ambivalence, poor adherence to treatment, and serious psychiatric or medical comorbidities. Given that only 10% of patients with substance use disorders actually receive specialized addiction treatment, it is clear that we need to help clinicians feel more comfortable assessing and treating substance use disorders in a range of clinical settings.

We put together a team of great scientists and educators who appreciate the complexities of addiction but also can simplify the material and make it accessible for people without specialized training. We hope that our little pocket guide will become a "go-to" reference tool for a wide range of clinicians—general psychiatrists, internists, family practitioners, pediatricians, emergency medicine physicians, residents and fellows from all specialties, medical students, allied professionals, and anyone who is fascinated by these devastating illnesses and committed to improving the lives of patients, and families of patients, with addiction.

This book is organized into three parts:

I. Fundamentals of Addiction
II. Substances and Behaviors
III. Treatment

Part I: Fundamentals of Addiction

The book begins with a brief overview of the neurobiology of addiction—our most current understanding of the complex neuroadaptations underlying the addictive process. We then present the landscape of addiction assessment and settings of care in the 21st century, as well as a brief treatment overview (more detail on treatment is provided in Part III). Finally, we discuss the DSM-5 diagnostic criteria of substance use disorder, as well as toxicology examinations.

Part II: Substances and Behaviors

The middle portion of the book addresses each class of drug of abuse, and a separate chapter provides discussion of behavioral addictions, with a focus on gambling disorder. Areas that are unique to specific classes of drugs or behaviors, such as recognition of intoxication or withdrawal syndromes and pharmacotherapy, are highlighted in this section.

Each chapter in Part II begins with a brief introduction about the specific substance class, including origins and trends of use, any specific populations that use the drug, and particular dangers about the drug; the chapters then proceed in the following general format:

1. Pharmacology
2. How to recognize intoxication
3. What to do about intoxication
4. How to recognize withdrawal
5. What to do about withdrawal
6. How to recognize addiction
7. What to do about addiction
8. Special issues with psychiatric comorbidities
9. Special issues with medical comorbidities
10. Special issues with specific populations

DSM-5 CRITERIA

For readers' ease of reference within each chapter in Part II, diagnostic criteria from the *Diagnostic and Statistical Manual of Mental Disorders*, Fifth Edition (DSM-5), are included for sub-stance-specific intoxication, withdrawal, and use disorders (as well as gambling disorder). Criteria sets contain the diagnostic criteria and listed subtypes and specifiers. The diagnostic criteria are reprinted with permission from the American Psychiatric Association. Readers are referred to DSM-5 for full diagnostic criteria sets, including subtype and specifier descriptions, coding notes, and recording procedures.

Part III: Treatment

The final section of the book provides detailed information on various aspects of addiction treatment that are generally applicable across most substance use disorders and behavioral addictions. Here we review evidence-based psychotherapies, 12-step programs, and lifestyle factors such as diet and exercise.

Acknowledgments

We hope that you will find this volume as helpful as it was gratifying for us to write. All three of us teach at Rutgers New Jersey Medical School, treat patients at University Hospital, and have been in touch several times a week for almost a year while working on this book—and that has been fun!

We are also deeply indebted to our colleagues, trainees, and students, who keep us intellectually honest and gave us wonderful ideas, encouragement, and feedback, sometimes in the form of tough love, throughout this project. Most of all, we would like to thank our amazing husbands, Lukas, Salvatore, and Anshu, who continue to suffer through, but lovingly endure and support, our psychiatric adventures year after year.

Petros Levounis, M.D., M.A.
Erin Zerbo, M.D.
Rashi Aggarwal, M.D.

PART

Fundamentals of Addiction

Neurobiology of Addiction

From Reward to Relief:
The Complex Neuroadaptations
Underlying Addiction

NATIONAL INSTITUTE ON
DRUG ABUSE

FOR decades, clinicians treating addiction have fought an uphill battle to get addiction recognized by the public, their patients, and even their medical colleagues as a medical illness rather than a moral failing. We have come a long way in helping people grasp that it is a disease that involves changes to an individual's brain. But there is still a long way to go in reducing the stigma of addiction, and it is partly the responsibility of researchers and clinicians in the addiction field to educate people on the complexity of this brain disease: The struggle waged by an individual with a substance use disorder is not just that of resisting the temptation of a pleasurable substance or of resisting the urge to "get high." Unfortunately, the past emphasis on dopamine-mediated brain reward processes could easily lead to such a simplified view.

The well-characterized actions of dopamine in the limbic reward system, including the circuits of the nucleus accumbens and the dorsal striatum, reflect only one phase (binge/

Reprinted with permission from the American Academy of Addiction Psychiatry (AAAP). This chapter was originally published as an article in the summer 2015 volume of *AAAP News*, p. 5.

intoxication) in the cycle of addiction. Recent advances in neuroimaging and genetics have greatly expanded and nuanced our understanding of the broader range of neuroadaptations occurring throughout the brain that characterize other phases of this complex disease. The acute dysphoria of withdrawal, for example, is now known to be mediated by circuits in basal forebrain areas and the extended amygdala (involving corticotropin-releasing factor, norepinephrine, and dynorphin). And drug craving and preoccupation involve executive functions mediated by glutamatergic circuits in the prefrontal cortex as well as circuits in the basolateral amygdala, hippocampus, and other regions involved in conditioned reinforcement and contextual information processing (Koob and Volkow 2010).

This broadened perspective has led to an understanding that negative reinforcement is just as important as positive reinforcement or reward in substance use disorders. The diminished sensitivity of reward neurocircuitry that is well known to occur in addicted individuals—for example, reduced expression of dopamine receptors (downregulation) in the striatum—is now known to be accompanied by greater recruitment of the stress or "anti-reward" systems that naturally act in opposition to reward, striving to maintain the motivational system in a state of balance (homeostasis) (Koob 2013). Thus, addicted individuals, for whom this motivational system is dysregulated, are driven to escape intolerable stress as much as by the need to experience reward. Moreover, "reward" has become so blunted that the drug is often not even experienced as pleasurable, merely as relief. The idea that people addicted to drugs take them to become intoxicated or get high (which implies pleasure) is thus very misleading.

The hedonic imbalance of addiction is further compounded by learned associations between drug reward—again, really relief—and environmental cues that have, over time, transformed the addicted person's world into a landscape of cues and triggers, like a video-game environment cunningly designed to pose the greatest challenge to his or her willpower at every turn. Additionally, we now know that the dopamine desensitization familiar in reward circuits also affects prefrontal circuits necessary for exerting self-control and following through with decisions. To further extend the video game metaphor, the resulting loss of self-control capacity is like replacing a functioning game controller with one whose buttons are unresponsive or stuck, steering the game-world persona in precisely the direction the player does not wish to go. Thus, even when people with addictions consciously choose to avoid drugs and the cues that lead them to drug use, they repeatedly find themselves acting against their intentions in a cycle of relapse.

In other words, the addicted person is really caught in a three-fold problem that cannot accurately be characterized as a temptation to get high on a pleasurable substance. Besides a physiologically based inability to experience healthy, non-drug behaviors as motivating, the addicted individual also experiences intolerable distress when without the drug, as a result of active recruitment of stress systems. What's more, even when the individual understands that this situation is untenable and opts to be rid of the drug and the trouble it is causing in his or her life, precisely the circuits necessary to follow through with that choice have been severely compromised. Addiction drastically reduces an individual's capacity to exert free will.

The good news is that we now have a fairly clear picture of the brain mechanisms underlying all phases of this process, and this will lead to new and improved treatment approaches over the coming years, as well as clinically useful biomarkers (Volkow et al. 2015). The bad news is that the wider world still does not understand the implications of having a brain disease that erodes something as basic as the ability to make and follow through with free choices and decisions. Perhaps because our culture places such a premium on freedom, people have trouble accepting that there exists a medical condition that actually erodes a person's capacity to act freely in their own best interests. This is the challenge of addiction both as a medical condition and as a cultural/social issue.

It has been a great struggle, unfolding for several decades, to change the public's perception of addiction from one of moral failure to the disease model now accepted by physicians. But to really get across that addiction is not merely a disease of the brain but specifically a condition in which fundamental motivational and self-control systems are damaged and cannot function properly may require challenging our culture's most core beliefs about personhood and the self.

References

Koob GF: Negative reinforcement in drug addiction: the darkness within. Curr Opin Neurobiol 23(4):559–563, 2013 23628232

Koob GF, Volkow ND: Neurocircuitry of addiction. Neuropsychopharmacology 35(1):217–238, 2010 19710631

Volkow ND, Koob G, Baler R: Biomarkers in substance use disorders. ACS Chem Neurosci 6(4):522–525, 2015 25734247

Addiction Assessment Across Settings of Care

Approaches for the Twenty-First Century

MIRELA FEURDEAN, M.D.

Magnitude of the Problem

Illicit drug use, which includes misuse of prescription pain-killers, has become a major societal problem in the United States and an "epidemic" worldwide. The most recent National Survey on Drug Use and Health (Substance Abuse and Mental Health Services Administration 2014) reported staggering numbers:

- An estimated 27 million Americans used illicit drugs in the month prior to the survey interview. This represents 10.2% of the U.S. population age 12 or older. The most common illicit drug used was marijuana (7.5%), followed by misuse of prescribed psychotherapeutic medication (1.6%) and cocaine (0.6%).
- An estimated 21.5 million Americans (or 8.1% of the population age 12 or older) were classified as having substance dependence or abuse in 2013. However, only 4.1 million received treatment, mostly at the level of a self-help group; less than 15% of them received treatment at a specialty facility.
- An estimated 66.9 million Americans (25.5%) used tobacco in the month before the survey.
- An estimated 2.8% of young adults (ages 18–25) misused pain relievers in 2014.

Who Is Called to Treat Addiction?

The statistics quoted in the previous section underscore the magnitude of the problem and the obvious issue of underdiagnosis and undertreatment. Given that almost 10% of the U.S. population struggles with drug addiction, physicians in all medical and surgical specialties are bound to meet these patients on a daily basis. However, more often than not, the addiction goes unaddressed; it will continue to lurk behind garden-variety health issues and will affect, unbeknownst to practitioners, the overall treatment outcome.

As a medical community, it is obvious that we must take a stance. Clinicians must start by becoming knowledgeable about drug intoxication and withdrawal. We must become alert to subtle and not so subtle signs of addiction and to comorbidities triggered or aggravated by specific drugs. Clinicians must also become skilled at taking an empathetic look at an uncomfortable situation. The undiagnosed patient may be in denial, and the conversations may become time-consuming; the discomfort of dealing with a negative attitude and the frustration of time-pressured visits should be balanced by empathy and strong skills in motivational interviewing (see Chapter 17, "Motivational Interviewing") in order to bring about a change in patients' health.

In the public conscience, psychiatry is viewed as the main medical specialty treating addiction, despite widespread statistics showing that only 30%–60% of patients with substance use disorder have a dual psychiatric diagnosis. Hence many patients remain outside the realm of the psychiatry service, and the effects of drug addiction on health permeate all medical and surgical subspecialties. The following subsections provide examples of common clinical scenarios that should trigger screening for substance use disorder.

PEDIATRICS AND ADOLESCENT MEDICINE

- Poor performance in school, reduced attention span, and memory deficits: screen for marijuana and inhalant use.
- Adolescents exposed to drugs early in life (most commonly, alcohol and marijuana) are several times more likely to develop a substance use disorder later in life, involving either the gateway drug or another substance, compared with adults who start using drugs after age 21.

- Hepatic steatosis on ultrasound or transaminitis: screen for alcohol use disorder before proceeding to exclude other causes of chronic liver disease.
- Chronic, recurrent nausea and vomiting without organic cause: screen for marijuana use.
- Anemia or unintentional weight loss: screen for malnutrition related to various substance use disorders.
- Chronic, resistant hypertension: screen for alcohol, tobacco, and cocaine use.
- Systolic heart failure: screen for alcohol and heroin use (toxic cardiomyopathy).
- Atrial fibrillation (paroxysmal or sustained): screen for alcohol and cocaine use. (Arrhythmia is commonly reversible if the drug is stopped.)
- Extensive dental cavities and chronic skin excoriations: screen for stimulant use (cocaine, methamphetamines).
- Skin rash and purpura: screen for cocaine use (cocaine-induced pseudovasculitis or leukocytoclastic vasculitis due to levamisole, a common adulterant in cocaine).
- Recurrent infections: screen for immunosuppression (HIV infection vs. agranulocytosis triggered by levamisole-contaminated cocaine).
- Peripheral neuropathy and central nervous system manifestations (e.g., forgetfulness, poor cognition and coordination): screen for prior inhalant use, alcohol use (cerebellar atrophy, Korsakoff psychosis), tobacco use (vascular dementia), cocaine use (reversible leukoencephalopathy due to levamisole), and HIV (HIV encephalopathy, cerebral infections, or lymphoma).
- Mood disorders: screen for history of substance use (e.g., "the crush" after cocaine use, protracted withdrawal syndrome from alcohol).
- Idiopathic chronic kidney disease: screen for heroin use (focal glomerulosclerosis) and HIV nephropathy.
- Poor libido and hypogonadism in men (e.g., chronic fatigue, testicular atrophy): screen for chronic opioid or illicit steroid use.
- Obesity, diabetes, hypertension, hyperlipidemia, or chronic obstructive pulmonary disease (COPD): classic medical pathology seen in primary care commonly involves some form of addiction, whether tobacco use disorder or behavioral addictions, that patients may not be

aware of. Good reflective listening skills will help diagnose and address these common barriers to successful treatment.

- Chronic noncancer-related pain: screen for personal and family history of substance use disorder, both essential in estimating the risk for iatrogenic addiction to painkillers; once medication for pain is prescribed, watch for potential misuse through history, state-sponsored prescription monitoring programs, and urine toxicology.
- Prescription medications: screen for chronic tobacco and alcohol use before prescribing certain medications (e.g., ketoconazole and metronidazole may induce a disulfiram-like reaction in patients who drink alcohol while taking these medications; tobacco enhances hepatic clearance of certain antipsychotics).

EMERGENCY AND HOSPITAL MEDICINE

- Hypertensive emergency: screen for cocaine, methamphetamine, and phencyclidine use.
- Acute vascular ischemia: screen for cocaine use. This is paramount to treatment, because selective β-blockers, otherwise a pillar of treatment for atherosclerotic coronary artery disease, would be harmful in the setting of cocaine-induced vasospasm.
- Asthma and COPD exacerbations: screen for drug inhalation (tobacco, cocaine, marijuana, inhalants).
- Acute respiratory failure: screen for cocaine and/or heroin use (noncardiogenic pulmonary edema, hypersensitivity pneumonitis—"crack lung").
- Acute renal failure: screen for cocaine use (acute rhabdomyolysis, renal cortical ischemia).
- Acute psychosis, seizures, or excessive sedation: screen for marijuana, cocaine, hallucinogen, alcohol, and sedative use.
- Acute delirium in the hospital: screen for substance use disorder (especially alcohol); benzodiazepines would be the treatment of choice for alcohol and sedative withdrawal, but they may trigger or aggravate delirium due to acute illness, so appropriate etiology must be established.

ANESTHESIOLOGY AND SURGICAL SPECIALTIES

- Preoperative evaluation should always include screening for recreational substance use disorder, as well as chronic opioid use for pain control.
- Drug screening is essential for prevention or treatment of potential withdrawal syndromes in the postoperative period; it also informs the choice of anesthetics (e.g., chronic cocaine users are at risk for hypertensive crisis if given local anesthesia containing epinephrine) and prescription of medications postoperatively.
- Medication metabolism can be impaired by concomitant illicit drug use:
  - Alcohol use increases tolerance for anesthetics and sedatives, whereas the presence of alcoholic liver disease will impair pharmacokinetics of drugs metabolized in the liver.
  - Tobacco stimulates the cytochrome P450 enzymatic system involved in the pharmacokinetics of many drugs, especially antipsychotics. Abstinence from tobacco for a few weeks, as is commonly advised preoperatively, may result in drug toxicity at doses on which the patient was previously stable.

OBSTETRICS AND GYNECOLOGY

- Amenorrhea or infertility in women: screen for cocaine and opiate use (hyperprolactinemia from drug-induced derangement in dopaminergic regulatory neurons).
- Pregnancy: screen for opiate and cocaine use (both are associated with pregnancy- and delivery-associated complications and neurobehavioral abnormalities in the newborn; both transfer into breast milk) and alcohol and inhalant use (teratogenic). Identification of substance use disorder should prompt treatment to maximize chances for a healthy pregnancy and a healthy infant.

GERIATRICS

Contrary to common belief, elderly people are at risk for substance use disorder that is difficult to diagnose in the absence of classic symptoms:

- Loneliness (nobody around to signal at-risk drinking) and retirement (no consequences at work to raise suspicion) can conceal early signs of substance use disorder.
- Trouble with alcohol in older people is sometimes mistaken for other conditions related to aging (e.g., a problem with balance or forgetfulness due to Alzheimer's dementia).

Many medications (prescription, over-the-counter, or herbs) can be dangerous or even deadly when mixed with alcohol.

General Examination: Clues for Substance Use Disorder

Discussed above, medical complications related to substance use disorders are a rather late stage in the diagnosis of addictive disease. It is more common to see patients in the hospital or in the office who do not have any of these medical complications, yet subtle findings on the review of systems and on clinical examination can suggest to the astute clinician the possibility of illicit drug use and trigger a thorough screening. These findings provide important opportunities for early diagnosis, and they apply to all subspecialties involved in outpatient care, including family practice, internal medicine and its subspecialties, gynecology, and dentistry. A few tips:

- History should always include a current list of medications. Presence of off-label use of medications (is such use medically plausible?) and chronic use or high doses of any psychotropic substances should prompt evaluation for substance use disorder.
- The clinician should address nonspecific complaints on the review of systems, such as unintentional weight loss (malnutrition due to most substance use, except marijuana), fatigue, and anhedonia (withdrawal from stimulants, chronic alcohol use).
- The physical examination can be very rich in findings for the trained eye, and particularly revealing to the clinician providing continuity of care. Changes in time, from one visit to the next, such as general deterioration of hygiene, attitude and mood, and physical health, are particularly telling.

- Other physical findings to look for:
  - *Skin:* venipuncture sites; jaundice; skin discoloration due to skin necrosis (levamisole) and palpable purpura (cocaine-induced vasculitis); petechiae, ecchymoses, telangiectasias (alcoholic liver disease), or stained fingers (marijuana and tobacco users); excessive perspiration (heroin); chronic excoriations or scabs (formication due to stimulants).
  - *Ear, nose, and throat:* rash around nose and mouth (inhalants); facial or lip burn (crack cocaine); nasal septal defects (sniffing cocaine); chronic rhinorrhea, loss of sense of smell, hoarseness (inhalants, cocaine, marijuana); bilateral swelling of parotids (alcohol); chronic conjunctival congestion (marijuana, inhalants); thrush (HIV, levamisole-induced agranulocytosis); dry mouth ("meth mouth"); discolored, worn-down teeth and extensive cavities, gingivitis, and periodontitis (stimulant-induced bruxism, "meth mouth"); dry lips, angular cheilitis, leukoplakia, and glossitis (nicotine-induced stomatitis); pupils very dilated (inhalants) or constricted (opioids).
  - *Lungs:* chronic congestion and cough, hemoptysis; wheezing and rales (tobacco, marijuana, inhalants, "crack lung").
  - *Cardiovascular:* hypertension—episodic or chronic (alcohol, tobacco, cocaine); tachycardia or arrhythmia (cocaine, alcohol, marijuana); heart murmurs in setting of constitutional symptoms (endocarditis from intravenous use of cocaine, heroin, and other drugs); weak pulses (tobacco is a strong risk factor for peripheral vascular disease).
  - *Abdomen:* hepatomegaly, splenomegaly, or ascites (cirrhosis due to alcohol, hepatitis B or C); chronic abdominal pain and constipation (opioids).
  - *Extremities:* chronic edema (alcoholic cirrhosis, nephrotic syndrome due to heroin or HIV-induced glomerulonephritis).
  - *Neurological:* fine tremors (alcohol, marijuana); peripheral neuropathy (alcohol, inhalants, vitamin deficiencies, HIV); poor coordination or abnormal cognitive function (alcohol).
  - *Psychiatric:* irritability, insomnia, or panic attacks (protracted alcohol withdrawal, sedative and marijuana

withdrawal); depression (withdrawal from stimulants, steroids); impairment of cognition (chronic alcohol and benzodiazepine use); hallucinations (hallucinogen persisting perception disorder).

For further information on DSM-5 diagnosis of substance-related disorders, as well as toxicology, see Chapter 3, "DSM-5 Diagnosis and Toxicology."

Does Screening Work?

Although subtle clinical findings should prompt evaluation for substance use disorder, this passive-reactive approach reaches too few patients, leaving the vast majority (who are asymptomatic) without treatment. Research focused on systematic population screening has found fair evidence that standardized questionnaires have acceptable accuracy and reliability in screening for drug use or misuse when applied to populations with a high prevalence of substance use disorder, but evidence of effectiveness is insufficient when applied to the general population (with a predictably lower prevalence of drug use or misuse) (U.S. Preventive Services Task Force 2015).

Many validated screening questionnaires, addressing various drugs and specific populations, are available online:

- For individuals age 18 or older: National Institute on Drug Abuse (NIDA) Quick Screen (one-question screening tool that takes the patient through use of multiple substances and can be used both online and in print; available at: www.drugabuse.gov/publications/resource-guide-screening-drug-use-in-general-medical-settings/nida-quick-screen)
- For adolescents under age 21: CRAFFT Screening Tool (available at: http://www.ceasar-boston.org/CRAFFT)
- For adults, the following screening tools are available:
  - Alcohol, Smoking and Substance Involvement Screening Test (ASSIST; available at: http://www.who.int/substance_abuse/activities/assist/en)
  - CAGE-AID (available a http://www.integration.samhsa.gov/images/res/CAGEAID.pdf)
  - Drug Abuse Screening Test (DAST)–20 (available at: http://www.emcdda.europa.eu/attachements.cfm/att_4094_EN_dast.html)

Proactive recruitment through screening has been shown to increase treatment recruitment rates, although treatment retention and complete abstinence remain poor despite stage-matched treatment interventions.

General Principles: How to Approach Patients

Approaching the subject of substance use with a patient who has not yet received an addiction diagnosis can be challenging, because many patients, especially active users, may not be forthcoming about their substance use disorder (e.g., denial, stigma associated with substance use).

The attitude of the physician in approaching the patient is essential: empathy and mutual trust are a must, and confidentiality of interview and physical findings must be affirmed clearly and reiterated at subsequent visits. The physician must be objective and nonjudgmental (e.g., state facts, help the patient interpret them) and respectful of a patient's autonomy (e.g., "I would like to discuss with you a concern....Is this okay with you?"). The patient's demeanor and body language may provide helpful clues with regard to his or her stage of change, as described by Prochaska and DiClemente (1984) and summarized in Table 2–1. Evaluation for psychological trauma (such as neglect, abandonment, and abuse in early life) and mental health issues is paramount, as is referral for treatment as necessary.

Patients' motivation to change depends on their stage of change; most undiagnosed patients are in the precontemplation and contemplation stages, but some may be prepared to take action. There appears to be no inherent motivation for patients to progress from one stage to the next, but an acute illness or early professional intervention may trigger change (Prochaska 2014).

Motivational interviewing capitalizes on these observations. The motivational interviewing approach blends empathy with active listening and patient-centered collaboration, in an effort to mobilize the patient's resources and motivation (desire, ability, reason, need, and commitment) to change, while supporting his or her autonomy and self-reliance. See Chapter 17, "Motivational Interviewing," for additional information.

The Screening, Brief Intervention, and Referral to Treatment (SBIRT) model of care combines systematic, universal

TABLE 2–1. Stages of change (Prochaska and DiClemente 1984)

Precontemplation: The patient is unaware or does not believe that there is a problem or may believe that there is a problem but is not considering changing behavior.

Contemplation: The patient is ambivalent about recognizing a problem and shies away from changing behavior.

Preparation: The patient is ready to work toward behavior change in the near future and develops a plan for change.

Action: The patient takes steps to implement specific behavior changes.

Maintenance: The patient works to maintain and sustain long-lasting behavior change.

Source. Adapted with permission from Arnaout B, Martino S: "Fundamentals of Motivation and Change," in *Handbook of Motivation and Change: A Practical Guide for Clinicians.* Edited by Levounis PL, Arnaout B. Washington, DC, American Psychiatric Publishing, 2010, p. 15. Used with permission. Copyright © 2010 American Psychiatric Publishing.

annual screening with motivational interviewing and stage-matched treatment on a continuum of patient care. (A practical description of SBIRT use in primary care is publicly available at www.sbirtoregon.org.) Studies have shown that the SBIRT model works best for addressing unhealthy alcohol use in patients seen by primary care physicians but is not effective at decreasing other drug use, such as cocaine use, marijuana use, or prescription drug misuse (Saitz et al. 2014).

The 5As Behavior Change model (Whitlock et al. 2002) can be adapted for any substance and/or behavior addiction counseling. The five steps are as follows:

1. *Assess* (beliefs, behaviors, and knowledge; readiness for change; data from physical examination and workup).
2. *Advise* (about health risks, benefits of change, treatment options).
3. *Agree* (on mutually accepted and realistic short- and long-term goals for behavior change).

4. *Assist* (in identifying and addressing personal barriers; providing resources, appropriate referrals, and regular follow-up)
5. *Arrange* (specific plan for follow up: office visits, phone calls, mailed reminders, and so forth)

The purpose of the stepwise approach in the 5As model is to have the patient develop and agree to a personal action plan that is then shared with the patient's practice team and social supports. To increase chances for success, the clinician should set realistic goals for brief encounters with patients at each stage of change and revisit these goals at subsequent visits. For more information, visit the U.S. Preventive Services Task Force Web page, "Behavioral Counseling Interventions: An Evidence-Based Approach": www.uspreventiveservicestaskforce.org/Page/Name/behavioral-counseling-interventions-an-evidence-based-approach.

Barriers to Care and How to Overcome Them

Attending to patients with substance use disorders is a difficult task, one that nonpsychiatrist physicians must undertake as well. Below are examples of common barriers to care encountered in clinical practice and a few tips on how to overcome them.

TIME-PRESSURED VISITS

Motivational interviewing (and other types of psychotherapeutic addiction treatments; see Part III, "Treatment") and coordination of care are time-consuming; ideally, addiction treatment should be integrated into a patient-centered medical home model, and physicians could delegate tasks accordingly to health care educators, social workers, nurses, and other health care professionals (O'Connor 2013).

DELAYED TREATMENT REWARDS

Addiction treatment is a long process; depending on the patient's stage of change, entering the maintenance phase may take years. Physicians should keep this in mind, tailor intervention to a patient's readiness to change, and adjust their own expectations accordingly. More importantly, maintaining a mutually collaborative relationship and a tone of hope without pressure to change will encourage the patient to come back and seek treatment when ready.

COMMON RELAPSES

Relapses are frequent and can feel like failure of treatment for both the patient and the physician. Clinicians as well as patients need to understand addiction as a chronic, relapsing neurochemical disease; accept relapses as part of the disease process; and maintain a positive outlook and hope for the long term (Rigotti 2012).

PSYCHOSOCIAL AND FINANCIAL ISSUES

Psychosocial and financial issues are commonly intertwined with substance use and are difficult to manage; unaddressed, they will undermine the effect of medical intervention. Patients need strong social work support embedded in the addiction treatment team.

KEY POINTS

Substance use disorders are very common yet largely underdiagnosed. Most physicians in medical or surgical specialties often encounter patients with addictions and could participate in their care.

Maintaining a high level of awareness, along with basic knowledge of the clinical presentation of intoxication and withdrawal and medical complications of substance abuse, is essential for diagnosis in the inpatient setting.

Empathy and reflective listening skills are essential tools for accurate diagnosis and successful intervention in the outpatient setting.

The nonpsychiatrist physician must work in concert with the social worker and the addiction specialist.

Primary care physicians can and should participate in the continuum of care for addiction: from screening and early diagnosis to outpatient detoxification and stabilization; reinforcing participation in specialty addiction treatment; posttreatment monitoring; and care coordination.

Behavioral addictions and the evolving domain of food addiction compound and color the treatment of common medical diseases.

References

O'Connor PG: Managing substance dependence as a chronic disease: is the glass half full or half empty? JAMA 310(11):1132–1134, 2013 24045739

Prochaska JO: Enhancing motivation to change, in The ASAM Principles of Addiction Medicine, 5th Edition. Edited by Ries RK, Fiellin DA, Miller SC, Saitz R. Philadelphia, Lippincott Williams & Wilkins, 2014, pp 833–844

Prochaska JO, DiClemente CC: The Transtheoretical Approach: Crossing Traditional Boundaries of Therapy. Homewood, IL, Dow Jones-Irwin, 1984

Rigotti NA: Strategies to help a smoker who is struggling to quit. JAMA 308(15):1573–1580, 2012 23073954

Saitz R, Palfai TP, Cheng DM, et al: Screening and brief intervention for drug use in primary care: the ASPIRE randomized clinical trial. JAMA 312(5):502–513, 2014 25096690

Substance Abuse and Mental Health Services Administration: Results from the 2013 National Survey on Drug Use and Health: Summary of National Findings (NSDUH Series H-48, HHS Publ No SMA 14-4863). Rockville, MD, Substance Abuse and Mental Health Services Administration, 2014. Available at: http://www.samhsa.gov/data/sites/default/files/NSDUHresultsPDFWHTML2013/Web/NSDUHresults2013.pdf. Accessed December 14, 2015.

U.S. Preventive Services Task Force: Final Update Summary: Drug Use, Illicit: Screening. Rockville, MD, U.S. Preventive Services Task Force, July 2015. Available at: http://www.uspreventiveservicestaskforce.org/uspstf/uspsdrug.htm. Accessed November 12, 2015.

Whitlock EP, Orleans CT, Pender N, Allan J: Evaluating primary care behavioral counseling interventions: an evidence-based approach. Am J Prev Med 22(4):267–284, 2002 11988383

DSM-5 Diagnosis and Toxicology

PETROS LEVOUNIS, M.D., M.A.

LINDSAY LYNCH, B.S.

DSM-5 Diagnosis

As discussed in Chapter 1 ("Neurobiology of Addiction"), the underlying neurobiology of addiction is fundamentally the same for a wide range of substances of abuse—and likely for the addictive behaviors as well. Likewise, the fifth edition of the *Diagnostic and Statistical Manual of Mental Disorders* (DSM-5; American Psychiatric Association 2013) contains diagnostic criteria for specific substance use disorders that are common across the 10 substance classes presented. Of note, the diagnoses of acute intoxication and withdrawal syndromes are specific to the substances used and will be presented later in Part II, "Substances and Behaviors," according to substance class. Part II also includes more in-depth discussion of specific substance use disorders.

DSM-5 defines *substance use disorder* as a problematic pattern of substance use leading to clinically significant impairment or distress manifested by at least 2 of the following 11 criteria occurring within a 12-month period. These criteria are organized memorably according to the mnemonic "The Wise Know: Decline Tender Loving Care And Respect Silver Hair" [Levounis 2015]). Corresponding criterion numerals (from any DSM-5 substance use disorder criteria set) are included for ease of reference:

1. **Physiology**
   - **T**olerance (Criterion 10)
   - **W**ithdrawal (Criterion 11)

2. **Core problem of addiction**
   - **K**nowledge of consequences, but continued use (Criterion 9)

3. **Internal preoccupation**
   - **D**esire to cut down (Criterion 2)
   - **T**ime—and a great deal of it—spent using and seeking the substance (Criterion 3)
   - **L**arger amounts or **L**onger use than intended (Criterion 1)
   - **C**ravings (Criterion 4)

4. **External consequences**
   - **A**ctivities given up (Criterion 7)
   - **R**ole obligations neglected (Criterion 5)
   - **S**ocial and interpersonal problems (Criterion 6)
   - **H**azardous use (Criterion 8)

5. **Current severity can be specified** in the diagnosis based on the number of criteria met:
   - *Mild:* Two to three criteria
   - *Moderate:* Four to five criteria
   - *Severe:* Six or more criteria

Toxicology

Drug testing, often referred to as *toxicology*, plays a critical role in evaluating and monitoring patients who use substances, regardless of whether they are abusing street drugs or using medications as prescribed. Drug testing has become an essential component of many areas of medical care, including substance abuse treatment and pain management. In addition, drug testing is used in forensics and the workplace, as well as clinical research and epidemiological studies.

DRUG TESTING SETTINGS

In clinical medicine, we appreciate that a perfect test does not exist, and thus, drug testing results are viewed in the context of a patient's history, physical examination, and other studies. In other settings, such as the criminal justice system or pre-employment screening, drug testing alone may be used to provide a "yes or no" answer to whether an individual has used certain drugs.

CLINICAL SETTINGS

In a clinical setting, drug testing is most commonly used to confirm or reinforce findings from the evaluation of a patient during the history and physical examination. Many clinicians currently prefer "point of care" immunoassays, which offer quick results. Often, a second, more sensitive and reliable test is selected to confirm the initial findings.

When selecting the best drug screening test to use, key questions to consider are the following:

- According to history and physical examination findings, which substance(s) has the patient most likely used?
- When did the patient most likely use the substances?
- Which screening test will detect the substance in the time frame between suspected drug use and presentation at the clinical center?
- What are the potential false-positive or false-negative results that will affect interpretation of the results?
- Should more than one screening test be used to confirm initial findings?

THE WORKPLACE AND CRIMINAL JUSTICE SYSTEM

Apart from clinical considerations, workplace or criminal justice system drug testing is concerned with an additional factor: the tests must be defensible in court. Strict chain of custody procedures must be maintained to ensure that the samples have not been altered or substituted. With this in mind, an initial screening test is used on-site, and then a second sample taken at the same time is sent out for a specific confirmation test. These confirmation tests are often specific to a single drug or drug metabolite. However, in clinical settings, such as a drug treatment center where the drug test is not intended to be defensible, a standard point of care test is sufficient.

AT HOME

With advances in technology, a variety of at-home drug testing kits have become available over the counter. On the one hand, home testing has the obvious advantage of privacy and convenience. On the other hand, testing through a third party offers the advantage of a clinician who has access to many resources and reliable testing methods, as well as training to interpret the results of a drug test and provide the patient with counseling about drug use. In general, at-home kits can and do work well, but they should not be used as a substitute for testing in a physician's office where a wider variety of more sensitive tests are available.

DRUG TESTING TYPES

IMMUNOASSAY SCREENING

When a quick result is needed (e.g., in an emergency department or a busy drug treatment clinic), a point of care immunoassay screening test is preferred. It is inexpensive and immediately indicates whether drugs or drug metabolites are present in a patient's urine. The assay is based on the concept of antibody binding. A color change that occurs when an antibody binds to its target denotes a positive result. In this case, the antibody target is either a drug or a drug metabolite.

Antibody targets must be present at certain concentrations to saturate enough of the antibodies for a positive color change to appear. Thus, when a clinician suspects drug use but the urine toxicology result is not positive, it may be helpful to send a second sample for analysis to confirm the presence or absence of a drug.

GAS CHROMATOGRAPHY/MASS SPECTROSCOPY TESTING

When the findings from an immunoassay must be confirmed, gas chromatography/mass spectroscopy (GC/MS) is often the best choice. In the time it takes for the samples to arrive and be processed at the specialized laboratories, clinicians rely on their point of care drug screening to direct a patient's assessment, diagnosis, and treatment. GC/MS is more expensive but provides more definitive answers and typically meets forensic standards. GC/MS testing can identify specific drugs in a variety of samples, including urine, blood, sweat, saliva, and hair. When GC/MS is used to confirm results of an immunoassay screening, it is preferable to collect the samples for the immunoassay and GC/MS at the same time, to prevent any confounding variables such as drug metabolism as a result of time elapsed between the two collections.

MASKING OF DRUG USE

With each advance in the technology of drug identification, a technique is often adapted to evade the new screening tool. This is often referred to as "masking." Some of the strategies used to mask drug use include the following:

- Switching to "designer drugs," which are synthesized with the goal of producing effects similar to those of the original drug while avoiding detection on standard drug screening tests.
- Substituting another person's urine as one's own when the urine collection is not directly observed for privacy reasons. Most point of care tests also measure the temperature of the sample in order to detect "imported" cold urine, but savvy individuals use devices to store the replacement urine at body temperature for the screening test.
- Using a fake penis (obviously, this technique works only for men!) when the urine collection is directly observed. The original false penis, called the "Whizzinator," is available in several skin tones, including white, tan, Latino, brown, and black.
- Taking diuretics in an attempt to clear a substance from one's urine quickly.
- Ingesting large amounts of water to dilute substances in one's urine to concentrations below detection levels. Most point of care tests also determine the specific gravity of the sample to detect grossly diluted urine.
- Ingesting large amounts of bicarbonate to alkalinize one's urine and thus decrease the elimination of amphetamines and methamphetamines.

With the constantly evolving struggle between more advanced drug testing and more advanced techniques to avoid drug detection, clinicians have adopted countermeasures to discourage the masking of drug use, such as testing samples other than urine. For example, testing hair samples can be particularly helpful if long-term drug use is suspected. A random rotating schedule of the type of sample collected decreases the risk of masking because the patient is unaware what specimen will be collected at any one time. Preparing to evade or circumvent drug detection in multiple body tissues is a very tall order.

SELECTING A SPECIMEN FOR TESTING

Certain tissues are better suited for detecting certain types of drugs, and different sample types provide information about a patient's drug use over different time frames. The most commonly used specimens include urine, blood, oral fluid, sweat, and hair. Each one of these drug testing methods has its own advantages and disadvantages.

URINE

Urine screening is the most commonly used method of drug testing because it is noninvasive, easy to obtain, inexpensive, and quick. Although the quantity of a drug or its metabolite cannot be accurately measured, urine samples can be assessed for the presence or absence of many drugs and their metabolites.

As discussed earlier, it is easy for urine samples to be altered or substituted. Techniques for measuring temperature, pH, creatinine, and specific gravity may be used to assess the reliability of a urine sample.

BLOOD

Blood samples allow for the accurate quantification of drugs and metabolites in a patient's system. Acquiring the sample is more invasive than urine collection and requires properly trained personnel for the venipuncture, but a quantitative result is sometimes needed for proper patient care. In blood samples, the presence of drugs or their metabolites can be detected for only a short window of time because most drugs are metabolized quickly by the body. Most blood samples require a few days to process; however, in an acute care setting, such as an emergency department or an intensive care unit, the results may be obtained quickly through the hospital's laboratory.

Blood samples are much more difficult than urine samples to alter or substitute and therefore provide more reliable information.

ORAL FLUID

In addition to being noninvasive, oral fluid collection does not have any of the privacy concerns associated with urine collection. Furthermore, drug concentrations in oral fluid correlate well with concentrations measured in blood samples. Oral fluid, however, can be easily contaminated by the collection technique or by whatever happens to be in the patient's mouth during or just before the time of collection.

Oral fluid samples are more difficult than urine samples for patients to alter and cannot be substituted because staff directly collect the sample or observe the patient while he or she collects the sample.

SWEAT

Using sweat to detect the use of drugs has become increasingly popular because it is noninvasive and allows for testing over a longer time. The individual to be tested wears a patch that detects drugs or drug metabolites excreted in sweat. The patch offers a good alternative for long-term monitoring because daily urine or blood collections are impractical.

The patch is difficult to tamper with because it can be applied only once. A noticeable alteration in the patch appears if it is removed and reapplied. Clinicians should always inspect the patch to make sure that it is in the same condition as when it was first applied.

HAIR

Hair samples are most often used in research studies or in settings where a forensically defensible sample is needed. Drugs and their metabolites are deposited into hair during the process of keratinization or directly deposited on hair from environmental contact. The hair sample is interpreted using segmental analysis. As the hair grows (approximately 1 cm per month), a history of the drugs is deposited in the hair. Drug use can be detected in the hair over long periods of time, up to 3 months; therefore, even if a patient abstains from his or her drug of choice leading up to the test, the hair sample will still show prior drug use. In conjunction with point of care testing such as urine toxicology examination, hair samples can provide a broad picture of a patient's chronic drug use. On the negative side, hair treatments, such as bleaching or dyeing, can alter the amounts of drug present in the hair, and environmental deposits in hair, such as through secondhand cannabis smoke, do not directly prove drug use. Furthermore, in clinical settings, hair testing is less useful because samples are sent out for analysis, which takes considerable time. In emergency departments, where patients may need immediate treatment for drug intoxication or withdrawal, hair testing is entirely impractical.

Hair is the easiest to collect and the most difficult to alter or substitute.

DETECTING COMMONLY USED SUBSTANCES

ALCOHOL

Screening tests for acute alcohol intoxication can determine the presence of alcohol and its metabolites in the body but cannot predict an individual's level of impairment. Therefore, even a person who may not present with severe impairment may still have dangerously high levels of alcohol in his or her body, especially if he or she has developed significant physiological tolerance to alcohol. Some screening tests routinely used to detect acute alcohol intoxication are the following:

- Blood alcohol concentration
- Breath alcohol concentration
- Oral fluid alcohol concentration
- Urine detection of ethyl glucuronide

Measurement of the concentration of alcohol in the blood is one of the first tests performed in the clinical setting but can detect alcohol in the body only for a few hours before it is cleared. Another method for detection of acute alcohol intoxication is the breath test, which law enforcement agents commonly use. For this test, the individual being tested exhales into a Breathalyzer, which measures the alveolar concentration of ethanol. Oral fluid is also used for rapid detection of ethanol in the saliva; however, it does not correlate well with blood levels of ethanol. In most states, the legal level of intoxication is 80 mg/dL.

A major problem with alcohol screening has been the short window of time during which alcohol can be detected in a patient's blood. Ethyl glucuronide is a direct metabolite of alcohol, which is present in the urine for up to 5 days depending on how much alcohol was consumed (Table 3–1). However, ethyl glucuronide is present in the urine even when a very small amount of alcohol is consumed or when an individual has used alcohol-containing products such as hand sanitizers or mouthwashes, resulting in false-positive results.

TABLE 3–1. Approximate urine toxicology detection limits

Substance	Time frame
Alcohol	6–12 hours
Alcohol (ethyl glucuronide)	4 days
Amphetamines/methamphetamines	2 days
Benzodiazepines (short-acting)	3 days
Benzodiazepines (long-acting)	30 days
Cocaine	3 days
Heroin (morphine)	2 days
Methadone	3 days
Marijuana (single use)	3 days
Marijuana (long-term heavy use)	30 days
Phencyclidine	7–21 days

Source. Adapted from Helander et al. 2009; Moeller et al. 2008.

CAFFEINE

Caffeine is not usually considered a drug of abuse because it is a commonly used and socially accepted stimulant. Although caffeine is potentially addictive, it has been shown to have some beneficial effects on several body systems. In rare instances, caffeine toxicity may be suspected in individuals presenting to the emergency department. Despite the growing presence of coffee and other caffeinated products all around the world, laboratory tests for caffeine are few and very rarely used. Caffeine toxicity is a relatively new concept in medicine and has not been fully described.

CANNABIS

The active ingredient in cannabis is delta-9-tetrahydrocannabinol (THC), but the inactive metabolite (11-*nor*-Δ^9-THC-9-carboxylic acid [THCA]) of the component is detected in drug screening tests. THC and THCA are lipophilic molecules and thus are stored in fat tissues. Because of its lipophilic nature, THCA can be detected in the urine of cannabis users for 30 days or more depending on the frequency of drug use. Although the federally mandated cutoff level for testing in the workplace is 50 ng/mL of THCA (and this same value is typically used in the clinical setting), THCA can be detected at levels of 15 ng/mL in urine screening tests if needed.

Patients undergoing chemotherapy may be prescribed synthetic THC (dronabinol) for the treatment of chemotherapy-related nausea and loss of appetite. If screened, these patients can have THCA in their urine.

HALLUCINOGENS

The hallucinogens are a group of substances that exert their effects through alterations in experience, perception, and consciousness. Some common hallucinogens that appear in the clinical setting include lysergic acid diethylamide (LSD), phencyclidine (PCP), and ketamine.

LSD. LSD is rapidly metabolized such that only small amounts of its metabolite N-desmethyl-LSD can be detected in the urine. Routine screening for LSD is rare because of the low specificity and high degree of cross-reactivity of the available immunoassays. Some of the substances that may cause a false-positive result for LSD are verapamil, haloperidol, metoclopramide, fluoxetine, amitriptyline, chlorpromazine, and risperidone.

PCP. Testing for PCP is mandated for federal employees and is often used in the clinical setting. PCP can be detected in the urine for up to 7 days after a single use and up to 21 days after repeated use. Blood screening is rarely performed because only low levels of PCP are found in the blood. Saliva testing is being explored as a screening method because levels of PCP are higher in saliva than in blood.

Ketamine. The metabolite of ketamine, norketamine, is not detected on routine urine screening tests but can be detected with specific immunoassays. Norketamine can be detected in urine for up to 3 days and for a week or more using GC/MS.

INHALANTS

Inhalants are gases or fumes that are inhaled with the intention of getting high. The major categories include volatile alkyl nitrites, nitrous oxide, volatile solvents, fuels, and anesthetics.

Inhalants are rapidly eliminated from the body and rarely detected in urine or blood.

OPIOIDS

The term *opioid* encompasses all substances that act like morphine in the body and includes natural, semisynthetic, and synthetic opioids.

- Natural opioids: morphine and codeine
- Semisynthetic opioids: hydromorphone, hydrocodone, oxymorphone, oxycodone, diacetylmorphine (heroin), and buprenorphine
- Synthetic opioids: methadone and fentanyl

When selecting a drug screening test, clinicians sometimes erroneously assume that an immunoassay for opioids will detect all opioids. Standard urine toxicology examinations reliably detect the naturally occurring opioids, morphine and codeine, as well as heroin because heroin quickly metabolizes into morphine. Standard tests, however, only occasionally have positive results for semisynthetic opioids, which require ordering specific tests for each semisynthetic opioid separately.

The confirmation cutoff value for morphine detection most commonly used in clinical settings is 300 ng/mL, whereas the cutoff value in the federal workplace is 2,000 ng/mL. The reasoning behind this dramatic difference is the potential for false-positive results. Ingestion of poppy seed muffins or poppy seed bagels can result in a urine level of 300 ng/mL for up to 48 hours after consumption, causing a false-positive result.

As diacetylmorphine (heroin) hydrolyzes to morphine, and before it loses both acetyl groups, it transiently becomes 6-monoacetylmorphine (6-MAM). This metabolite is uniquely found in the metabolism of heroin and therefore allows the clinician to differentiate heroin use from morphine or codeine use. However, 6-MAM rapidly hydrolyzes further into morphine and can be detected in urine samples for only up to 8 hours after heroin use.

Confirmatory testing for specific semisynthetic opioids is extremely complicated because many of the prescribed opioids are minor metabolites of other opioids. For example, for a patient who is prescribed hydrocodone, hydromorphone is a metabolite that will be detected in his or her urine. In the case of methadone, the screening immunoassay has very little cross-reactivity with the other opioids.

SEDATIVES, HYPNOTICS, AND ANXIOLYTICS

The major groups of substances within the sedative, hypnotic, and anxiolytic drug class include the barbiturates, the benzodiazepines, and a newer group of drugs termed the *nonbenzodiazepines*. The nonbenzodiazepines (zolpidem, zaleplon, eszopiclone), sometimes also called the "z-drugs," act somewhat similarly to benzodiazepines and are used in the treatment of insomnia.

Barbiturates. Drug screening for barbiturates is relatively straightforward because the urine immunoassays are specific. The short-acting barbiturates can be detected in urine for 1–4 days, and phenobarbital can be detected for several weeks.

Benzodiazepines. Much like with the semisynthetic opioids, interpreting the urine immunoassays for benzodiazepines is complicated by the variety of drugs and their metabolites. The cutoff used in the clinical setting is 200 or 300 ng/mL, but only high doses of the drugs can be detected at this level, whereas most therapeutic doses will not give a positive urine toxicology examination result.

Nonbenzodiazepines. The routine benzodiazepine immunoassays will not detect zolpidem, zaleplon, or eszopiclone.

STIMULANTS

Within the class of stimulants, the two major drugs of clinical significance are cocaine and the amphetamines, including the methamphetamines. Unfortunately, amphetamines have high levels of cross-reactivity with several other similar compounds, and the screening tests for amphetamines have a high incidence of false-positive results. Compounds eliciting a false-positive result for amphetamine include the following:

- Nasal decongestants such as phenylpropanolamine, pseudoephedrine, and L-methamphetamine
- Appetite suppressants containing ephedrine or phentermine

- L-Amphetamine/D-amphetamine, a common medication for attention-deficit/hyperactivity disorder, which is metabolized to amphetamine

The screening test for cocaine targets the major metabolite of cocaine: benzoylecgonine. Benzoylecgonine is a specific metabolite of cocaine and can be detected in urine for up to 2–3 days after cocaine use. It is not possible to differentiate between cocaine hydrochloride (powdered) and crack cocaine with the urine immunoassay. The urine immunoassays for benzoylecgonine have not shown false-positive results with other drugs.

TOBACCO

Screening for tobacco use is not very common in a clinical care setting but is commonly used by insurance companies to evaluate individuals for policies. Oral fluid screening has become increasingly popular for tobacco screening. Major metabolites of nicotine include cotinine, anabasine, and nornicotine. To differentiate between cigarette use and other sources of nicotine, anabasine or nornicotine may be targeted in the immunoassay because these metabolites are not generated by the nicotine patch or nicotine gum.

OTHER (OR UNKNOWN) SUBSTANCES

Emerging drugs of abuse not detected in routine screening tests include the bath salts and the synthetic cannabinoids. Bath salts are synthetic variants of a compound called cathinone, which is structurally identical to amphetamine with the addition of one single carbonyl bond to the beta carbon. A variety of synthetic cathinone compounds exist, and most of them are not detected on routine urine screening. One of the more prevalent synthetic cathinones in the United States is 3,4-methylenedioxypyrovalerone (MDPV). MDPV is not detected on routine urine screening but can be detected in urine within 20 hours of use with GC/MS. Routine drug screening cannot detect the synthetic cannabinoids; however, new assays are being developed to target their metabolites.

Anabolic-androgenic steroids are banned in all major professional sports, and athletes are regularly screened. The primary method for detecting steroid use is with urine screening tests. Anabolic-androgenic steroids undergo significant biotransformation in the liver and are then excreted in the urine. Most of these substances are metabolized by similar mechanisms and therefore have common metabolites, which are then detected in screening tests. This common final metabolic pathway makes detection of anabolic-androgenic steroids relatively straightforward—but makes determination of which substance initially used nearly impossible.

KEY POINTS

The DSM-5 diagnosis of substance use disorders is based on physiology, continued use despite knowledge of ongoing problems, internal preoccupation, and external consequences.

An ethyl glucuronide urine test can detect alcohol use for several days after last ingestion.

Delta-9-tetrahydrocannabinol can be detected in urine for 30 days or more in heavy cannabis users.

The routine benzodiazepine immunoassays will not detect zolpidem, zaleplon, or eszopiclone.

Ingestion of poppy seed muffins or bagels may cause a false-positive urine test result for codeine and morphine. A positive 6-monoacetylmorphine (6-MAM) test result is pathognomonic for heroin use—no other substance will have a positive 6-MAM test result.

Standard opioid tests typically give negative results for semisynthetic and synthetic opioids. Amphetamine tests often give false-positive results.

Cocaine is cocaine—cocaine tests are unlikely to give either false-positive or false-negative results.

Bath salts and synthetic cannabinoids do not show up in routine drug screening.

References

American Psychiatric Association: Diagnostic and Statistical Manual of Mental Disorders, 5th Edition. Arlington, VA, American Psychiatric Association, 2013

Helander A, Böttcher M, Fehr C, et al: Detection times for urinary ethyl glucuronide and ethyl sulfate in heavy drinkers during alcohol detoxification. Alcohol Alcohol 44(1):55–61, 2009 18971292

Levounis P: The wise know: decline tender loving care and respect silver hair. Acad Psychiatry 39(2):235, 2015 25488903

Moeller KE, Lee KC, Kissack JC: Urine drug screening: practical guide for clinicians. Mayo Clin Proc 83(1):66–76, 2008 18174009

Additional Readings

Galanter M, Kleber HD, Brady KT: The American Psychiatric Publishing Textbook of Substance Abuse Treatment, 5th Edition. Washington, DC, American Psychiatric Association Publishing, 2015

Levounis P, Herron AJ: The Addiction Casebook. Washington, DC, American Psychiatric Publishing, 2014

Renner JA, Levounis P: Handbook of Office-Based Buprenorphine Treatment of Opioid Dependence. Washington, DC, American Psychiatric Publishing, 2011

Ries RK, Fiellin DA, Miller SC, et al (eds): The ASAM Principles of Addiction Medicine, 5th Edition. Philadelphia, PA, 2014

Shults TF: Medical Review Officer Handbook, 9th Edition. Research Triangle Park, NC, Quadrangle Research, 2009

PART II

Substances and Behaviors

CHAPTER 4

Alcohol

FAYE CHAO, M.D.

NAUMAN ASHRAF, M.D.

ALCOHOL is one of the oldest psychoactive substances known, with use dating back 10,000–12,000 years. Alcohol use is nearly ubiquitous in modern times, and in the United States, lifetime exposure approaches 90%. Because of alcohol's legal status and social acceptability, a common misconception is that alcohol is somehow a less harmful substance than street drugs such as heroin and cocaine. However, the misuse of alcohol is very common.

- Lifetime prevalence of any alcohol use disorder is 30.3% (Hasin et al. 2007).
- Prevalence of alcohol use is highest among young adults.
- Alcohol is involved in about 40% of crimes of violence (Greenfield 1998).
- Alcohol is involved in about 40% of motor vehicle accidents in the United States, more than any other substance (Greenfield 1998).
- It has been estimated that in the United States, the annual cost of alcohol-related problems—from loss of workplace productivity, health care expenses, and criminal justice issues—is in excess of $200 billion (Centers for Disease Control and Prevention 2014).

Pharmacology

PHARMACOKINETICS

Ingestible alcohol (ethanol) is the product of the fermentation process. Alcohol is most often administered orally, although inhaled and rectal routes of administration also have been reported. It is a water-soluble molecule that is absorbed from the stomach, small intestine, and colon, and rate of absorption is determined by gastric emptying time and presence of food in the small intestine.

A standard drink is defined as any drink that contains 14 g of pure alcohol. Most alcoholic beverages have an alcohol content that ranges between 3% and 70%. In the United States, alcoholic beverages are usually labeled with a proof, which equals twice the alcohol by volume (e.g., 80 proof=40% alcohol by volume). Typically, 12 oz of beer=8 oz of malt liquor=5 oz of wine=1.5 oz of hard liquor (e.g., vodka, tequila, whiskey).

Blood alcohol level (BAL) is the amount of alcohol present in 100 mL (or 1 dL) of blood (e.g., BAL of 0.08=0.08 g/dL=80 mg/dL or mg%). BAL is determined by body weight and gender. When body weights are equivalent, women have 20%–25% higher BALs after ingestion of the same amount of alcohol than do men; this may be a result of less gastric metabolism in women, because levels are not different when the alcohol is administered intravenously.

Metabolism is primarily enzymatic and is carried out via zero-order kinetics (Figure 4–1). BAL decreases by about 0.02 g/dL/hour.

PHARMACODYNAMICS

Alcohol has several different effects on neurotransmitter systems. It does not directly agonize any one receptor but rather modulates transmission at different targets. Alcohol enhances activity at the γ-aminobutyric acid A (GABA$_A$) receptor (may be due to changes in presynaptic release) and inhibits activity at the N-methyl-D-aspartate (NMDA) receptor. This increase in inhibitory signaling and decrease in excitatory signaling are what mediates acute intoxication and the sedative effects of alcohol. Also, decreases in glutamate can lead to increased dopamine in the nucleus accumbens (thus enhancing the rewarding effects of alcohol), and decreases in glutamate in the prefrontal cortex (which controls complex cognitive behaviors and decision making) lead to cognitive deficits and errors in judgment.

Alcohol also increases serotonin activity at the serotonin type 3 (5-HT$_3$) receptor. In animal studies, 5-HT$_3$ antagonism blocks rats' ability to distinguish between alcohol and saline,

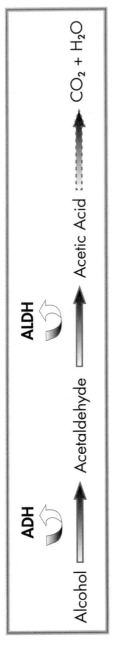

FIGURE 4–1. Alcohol metabolism.

Initially, alcohol is converted by alcohol dehydrogenase (ADH) into acetaldehyde. Acetaldehyde is further broken down into acetic acid by aldehyde dehydrogenase (ALDH).

Alcohol

41

so this receptor may be responsible for some of the subjective effects.

Additional effects include the following:

- Increased or decreased activity at nicotinic receptors. These receptors are found in structures that make up the reward pathway (nucleus accumbens, ventral tegmental area, and prefrontal cortex).
- Increased release of β-endorphin
- Increased corticotropin-releasing factor
- Unclear effect at the cannabinoid type 1 (CB_1) receptor. In studies, CB_1 antagonism or knockouts produce decreased alcohol preference and prevent increase in dopamine in the nucleus accumbens.

How to Recognize Intoxication

Alcohol is a central nervous system (CNS) depressant, and effects vary depending on dose.

- Initial effects (BAL=20–99 mg%): disinhibition, relief of anxiety, increased talkativeness, and feelings of confidence and euphoria
- Later effects (BAL=100–200 mg%): impairment of judgment and reaction time, increased emotional outbursts, and ataxia
- Even later effects (BAL>200 mg%): very obvious intoxication, nausea, vomiting, marked ataxia, severe dysarthria, amnesia, hypothermia

DSM-5 criteria for alcohol intoxication (Box 4–1; American Psychiatric Association 2013) are included for reference.

Box 4–1.   Diagnostic Criteria for Alcohol Intoxication

A. Recent ingestion of alcohol.
B. Clinically significant problematic behavioral or psychological changes (e.g., inappropriate sexual or aggressive behavior, mood lability, impaired judgment) that developed during, or shortly after, alcohol ingestion.
C. One (or more) of the following signs or symptoms developing during, or shortly after, alcohol use:

1. Slurred speech.
2. Incoordination.
3. Unsteady gait.
4. Nystagmus.
5. Impairment in attention or memory.
6. Stupor or coma.

D. The signs or symptoms are not attributable to another medical condition and are not better explained by another mental disorder, including intoxication with another substance.

TOLERANCE

Tolerance can develop to all effects of alcohol, and the degree of tolerance can be inferred from the patient's clinical presentation and BAL (e.g., a patient who shows withdrawal symptoms at a BAL of 150 mg% has a high tolerance).

OBTAINING THE HISTORY

The clinician should determine alcohol use (type of alcohol, amount, method of use, last use) and any other concurrent drug use. Alcohol can potentiate the effects of other CNS depressants such as benzodiazepines; it also can inhibit cocaine metabolism and form a more potent and toxic metabolite with cocaine called cocaethylene. The clinician also should obtain collateral information from family, friends, or medical records.

What to Do About Intoxication

Treatment of alcohol intoxication is mainly supportive.

- Vital signs should be frequently monitored.
- Care should be taken to protect the airway (particularly if the patient is unconscious).
- Intravenous fluids are often necessary.
- Intravenous thiamine and/or glucose may be given as well; however, thiamine must be administered *before* glucose because large doses of intravenous glucose can precipitate encephalopathy in a patient with subclinical thiamine deficiency.
- The BAL should be measured because this can help indicate a patient's tolerance and likelihood of developing withdrawal symptoms.

- Electrolyte imbalances, particularly hypomagnesemia, are also quite common in alcohol use disorders, and a basic metabolic panel is frequently recommended.
- A urine toxicology screen can indicate if a patient has ingested any other substances that are contributing to the intoxication and need to be addressed.
- Hemodialysis may be required in severe cases (e.g., BAL>400 mg% in an unresponsive person).

How to Recognize Withdrawal

The onset of alcohol withdrawal is 6–48 hours after the last drink, and withdrawal typically peaks around 24 hours after the last drink. Withdrawal symptoms include the following:

- Tremulousness
- Diaphoresis
- Insomnia with or without nightmares
- Elevated blood pressure and heart rate
- Nausea or vomiting, loss of appetite
- Headache
- Anxiety
- Irritability

Withdrawal can be measured by the Clinical Institute Withdrawal Assessment for Alcohol Scale, Revised (CIWA-Ar; Sullivan et al. 1989), a 10-item scale used to assess the severity of alcohol withdrawal and that can help guide treatment (Table 4–1). DSM-5 criteria for alcohol withdrawal (Box 4–2) are included for reference.

Alcohol withdrawal also can progress to more severe syndromes such as withdrawal seizures and delirium tremens (DTs). Withdrawal seizures occur in about 3% of those with physiological dependence on alcohol and arise within the first 12–48 hours after the last drink. Patients experience generalized tonic-clonic seizures, and in about 3% of cases, patients will develop status epilepticus. DTs generally occurs within 48–72 hours after the last drink but may arise as far out as 1 week from last use. About 5% of patients with physiological dependence on alcohol will develop DTs. It is characterized by delirium, tremors, autonomic instability (fever, tachycardia, hypertension), agitation (but also can be stuporous), and hallucinations (often tactile and/or visual). Untreated, DTs has about a 20% mortality rate.

TABLE 4–1. Items rated in the Clinical Institute Withdrawal Assessment for Alcohol Scale, Revised (CIWA-Ar)

1. **Nausea/Vomiting**—none (0); mild nausea without vomiting (1); intermittent nausea with dry heaving (4); constant nausea, frequent dry heaving, vomiting (7)

2. **Tremor** *(observe with patient's arms extended/fingers spread apart)*—none (0); not visible but felt fingertip to fingertip (1); moderate with arms extended (4); severe even with arms not extended (7)

3. **Paroxysmal sweats** *(observe)*—none (0); barely perceptible sweating, palms moist (1); beads of sweat on forehead (4); drenching sweats (7)

4. **Anxiety** *(question and observe)*—none (0); mildly anxious (1); moderately anxious or guarded (such that anxiety is inferred) (4); level equivalent to acute panic states, as seen in severe delirium or acute schizophrenic reactions (7)

5. **Agitation** *(observe)*—none (0); somewhat more than normal activity level (1); moderately fidgety/restless (4); paces back and forth during most of interview, thrashing about in bed (7)

6. **Tactile disturbances** *(question and observe)*—none (0); very mild itching, pins and needles, burning or numbness (1); mild itching, pins and needles, burning or numbness (2); moderate itching, pins and needles, burning or numbness (3); moderately severe hallucinations (4); severe hallucinations (5); extremely severe hallucinations (6); constant hallucinations (7)

7. **Auditory disturbances** *(question and observe)*—none (0); very mild harshness or ability to frighten (1); mild harshness or ability to frighten (2); moderate harshness or ability to frighten (3); moderately severe hallucinations (4); severe hallucinations (5); extremely severe hallucinations (6); constant hallucinations (7)

8. **Visual disturbances** *(question and observe)*—none (0); very mild light/color sensitivity (1); mild sensitivity (2); moderate sensitivity (3); moderately severe hallucinations (4); severe hallucinations (5); extremely severe hallucinations (6); constant hallucinations (7)

9. **Headache/Fullness in head** *(question and rate severity—do not rate dizziness/lightheadedness)*—none (0); very mild (1); mild (2); moderate (3); moderately severe (4); severe (5); very severe (6); extremely severe (7)

10. **Orientation/Clouding of sensorium** *(ask day, locations, who the interviewer is; have patient count forward by 3's)*—oriented and able to do serial additions (0); cannot do serial additions or uncertain about date (1); disoriented to date by no more than 2 calendar days (2); disoriented to date by more than 2 days (3); disoriented to place and/or person (4)

Scoring (points)

0–9: very mild withdrawal

10–15: mild withdrawal

16–20: modest withdrawal

21–67: severe withdrawal

Source.   Adapted from Sullivan et al. 1989.

Box 4–2.   Diagnostic Criteria for Alcohol Withdrawal

A. Cessation of (or reduction in) alcohol use that has been heavy and prolonged.

B. Two (or more) of the following, developing within several hours to a few days after the cessation of (or reduction in) alcohol use described in Criterion A:

  1. Autonomic hyperactivity (e.g., sweating or pulse rate greater than 100 bpm).

  2. Increased hand tremor.

3. Insomnia.
4. Nausea or vomiting.
5. Transient visual, tactile, or auditory hallucinations or illusions.
6. Psychomotor agitation.
7. Anxiety.
8. Generalized tonic-clonic seizures.

C. The signs or symptoms in Criterion B cause clinically significant distress or impairment in social, occupational, or other important areas of functioning.

D. The signs or symptoms are not attributable to another medical condition and are not better explained by another mental disorder, including intoxication or withdrawal from another substance.

Specify if:
With perceptual disturbances

What to Do About Withdrawal

Withdrawal can be managed in several different settings, including outpatient settings, inpatient detoxification units, and medical units. In each of these settings, treatment primarily involves using benzodiazepines to control withdrawal symptoms. Medication can be given by mouth, intramuscularly, or intravenously, depending on the severity of withdrawal. Once the patient is comfortable, the dosage of the benzodiazepine is gradually tapered over time down to zero. The slower the medication is tapered, the more comfortable the patient will be once the medication is discontinued. The total daily dose should be decreased by no more than 20% with each dosage change.

No single benzodiazepine has been proven to be more effective than another in managing withdrawal. In general, the longer-acting agents such as chlordiazepoxide, clonazepam, and diazepam are preferred because they may provide a smoother withdrawal course with fewer breakthrough symptoms. However, their long half-lives result in an increased risk for oversedation. Somewhat shorter-acting agents such as lorazepam may be preferable in elderly patients because they are less likely to accumulate on repeated administration; lorazepam is also preferred for patients with liver disease because it is renally excreted, and metabolism is not affected by liver impairment. If intramuscular medication is needed, lorazepam is most commonly used (intramuscular diazepam should be avoided because of erratic absorption via this route). Both diazepam and lorazepam may be used intravenously. If a switch from one benzodiazepine to another is necessary, an equivalency table can be helpful (Table 4–2).

TABLE 4–2. Equivalency doses and half-lives for commonly used benzodiazepines

Benzodiazepine	Half-life (hours)	Equivalent dose (oral, mg)
Chlordiazepoxide	5–100 (due to active metabolites)	25
Lorazepam	10–20	1
Diazepam	20–50	10
Clonazepam	20–40	0.5

Two approaches for dosing regimens are commonly used for medically managed withdrawal, each with its own advantages and disadvantages: symptom-triggered and fixed dosing regimens.

With *symptom-triggered management,* medication is given based on the presence of signs and symptoms of withdrawal; usually, the CIWA-Ar scale is used to measure the severity of the withdrawal. This method decreases the risk of oversedation and may allow a patient to complete detoxification faster with less overall medication. However, for those patients with very high tolerance or at risk for severe withdrawal syndromes, this method runs the risk of underdosing the patient because withdrawal symptoms can progress in severity faster than the ability to control them with as-needed dosing.

With a *fixed dosing regimen,* medication is given on a predetermined dosing regimen based on the patient's estimated tolerance. As-needed doses often are made available to account for underdosing of the regimen; however, the patient's tolerance may be overestimated, and the patient may become sedated. For patients at risk for severe withdrawal, fixed dosing regimens may be preferable because the risk of harm from DTs or seizures is greater than the risk from sedation. One way to mitigate the risk of sedation from a fixed dosing regimen is to give smaller, more frequent doses throughout the day. For example, although the long half-life of chlordiaz-epoxide would technically allow for once-a-day dosing, dividing the total daily dose into every 4 or 6 hours allows for more frequent contact with staff and the ability to hold doses should the patient start to appear sedated.

Examples of both regimens are as follows:

- A sample symptom-triggered regimen might be chlordiaz-epoxide 25 mg orally every 2 hours as needed (CIWA-Ar scale score≥10).
- A sample fixed dosing regimen might be the following:
  - Chlordiazepoxide 25 mg orally every 4 hours (6 doses)
  - Decreased to chlordiazepoxide 20 mg orally every 4 hours (6 doses)
  - Then decreased to chlordiazepoxide 15 mg orally every 4 hours (6 doses)
  - Finally decreased to chlordiazepoxide 10 mg orally every 4 hours (6 doses)
  - In addition, chlordiazepoxide 25 mg orally every 4 hours as needed (CIWA-Ar scale score≥10) may be ordered.

Comfort medications for symptomatic relief may be necessary as well.

- For nausea, metoclopramide 10 mg orally or intramuscularly three times a day as needed or ondansetron 4 mg orally or intramuscularly three times a day as needed may be used.
- For pain or headache, ibuprofen 600 mg orally every 6 hours as needed or acetaminophen 650 mg orally every 6 hours as needed may be used, but clinicians should be careful in selecting an appropriate analgesic because patients with alcohol use disorder frequently have medical comorbidities that would prohibit the use of one or another of these medications (e.g., liver dysfunction, history of gastrointestinal bleeding).
- Patients withdrawing from alcohol very frequently have insomnia (resulting from autonomic arousal) and night-mares (caused by rapid eye movement rebound), and sleep aids such as trazodone 50 mg orally every night at bedtime as needed, diphenhydramine 50 mg orally every night at bedtime as needed, or hydroxyzine 50 mg orally every night at bedtime as needed can help.

- Diphenhydramine and hydroxyzine also can be given during the daytime if the patient is experiencing anxiety; gabapentin is another frequently used medication for anxiety during withdrawal, and some evidence indicates that it may help curb addiction as well.
- Finally, loperamide 2 mg orally every 2 hours as needed for diarrhea is often used.

The development of withdrawal seizures may require that the benzodiazepine dose be increased or the taper schedule slowed down. If a patient is being detoxified as an outpatient, the development of seizures indicates that a higher level of care is necessary, and she or he should be admitted to either an inpatient detoxification unit or a medical unit for closer monitoring. If the patient is already admitted to a unit, a neurology consultation would be prudent, especially if the patient has other risk factors for seizures (history of falls and other accidents are common in this population). The seizures themselves are usually self-limited, but the patient will need monitoring in the postictal period. However, 3% of patients who have withdrawal seizures will develop status epilepticus, which is a medical emergency. Some evidence indicates that starting an antiepileptic drug such as valproic acid or levetiracetam at the outset of detoxification in patients with a history of withdrawal seizures may help mitigate the risk of future seizures.

DTs is considered a medical emergency and generally requires treatment in an intensive care unit setting. Patients require large doses of intravenous benzodiazepines (e.g., lorazepam, diazepam) and sometimes require the addition of an intravenous barbiturate (e.g., phenobarbital). Additionally, supportive care is provided such as intravenous fluids, correction of any electrolyte abnormalities, intravenous thiamine if necessary, 5% dextrose if necessary, and small amounts of antipsychotics for agitation.

How to Recognize Addiction

As with any patient encounter, a thorough history is essential. Many patients may be experiencing guilt over their substance use and have had negative experiences with the medical community because of the stigma of addiction. The initial encounter is important in establishing rapport and fostering openness in the relationship. The attitude of the interviewer should be nonjudgmental, curious, respectful, and professional.

NIAAA DEFINITIONS

The National Institute on Alcohol Abuse and Alcoholism (2010) defines at-risk drinking as follows:

- Men: >4 drinks/day, >14 drinks/week
- Women: >3 drinks/day, >7 drinks/week
- One drink=12 oz beer or wine cooler, 5 oz wine, 2–3 oz cordials or liqueur, or 1.5 oz 80-proof spirits

Practitioners can begin their alcohol screening process with one question:

- "Do you sometimes drink beer, wine, or other alcoholic beverages?"

If the patient's answer is "No," alcohol screening can be concluded for this visit. If the answer is "Yes," an additional quick screen follows:

- "How many times in the past year have you had five (for men)/four (for women) or more drinks in 1 day?"

Any nonzero answer should prompt the provider to begin more in-depth screening for alcohol misuse with the instruments discussed later in this section.

DSM-5 criteria for alcohol use disorder (Box 4–3) are included for reference.

Box 4–3.   Diagnostic Criteria for Alcohol Use Disorder

A. A problematic pattern of alcohol use leading to clinically significant impairment or distress, as manifested by at least two of the following, occurring within a 12-month period:

1. Alcohol is often taken in larger amounts or over a longer period than was intended.
2. There is a persistent desire or unsuccessful efforts to cut down or control alcohol use.
3. A great deal of time is spent in activities necessary to obtain alcohol, use alcohol, or recover from its effects.

4. Craving, or a strong desire or urge to use alcohol.
5. Recurrent alcohol use resulting in a failure to fulfill major role obligations at work, school, or home.
6. Continued alcohol use despite having persistent or recurrent social or interpersonal problems caused or exacerbated by the effects of alcohol.
7. Important social, occupational, or recreational activities are given up or reduced because of alcohol use.
8. Recurrent alcohol use in situations in which it is physically hazardous.
9. Alcohol use is continued despite knowledge of having a persistent or recurrent physical or psychological problem that is likely to have been caused or exacerbated by alcohol.
10. Tolerance, as defined by either of the following:
    a. A need for markedly increased amounts of alcohol to achieve intoxication or desired effect.
    b. A markedly diminished effect with continued use of the same amount of alcohol.
11. Withdrawal, as manifested by either of the following:
    a. The characteristic withdrawal syndrome for alcohol (refer to Criteria A and B of the criteria set for alcohol withdrawal).
    b. Alcohol (or a closely related substance, such as a benzodiazepine) is taken to relieve or avoid withdrawal symptoms.

Specify if:
In early remission
In sustained remission

Specify if:
In a controlled environment

Specify current severity:
Mild: Presence of 2–3 symptoms.
Moderate: Presence of 4–5 symptoms.
Severe: Presence of 6 or more symptoms.

THE CAGE

The CAGE questions are frequently used as a screening tool to identify patients who may be engaging in problematic drinking behaviors and merit further investigation. These four questions make up the CAGE questionnaire:

1. Have you ever felt you should **C**ut down on your drinking?
2. Have people **A**nnoyed you by criticizing your drinking?

3. Have you ever felt bad or **G**uilty about your drinking?
4. Have you ever had a drink first thing in the morning to steady your nerves or to get rid of a hangover (**E**ye opener)?

THE AUDIT-C

The U.S. Preventive Services Task Force has recommended that all patients 18 years or older be screened for alcohol misuse and recommends screening tools such as the Alcohol Use Disorders Identification Test (AUDIT). The AUDIT is a 10-item paper-and-pencil test that can be administered if a patient scores 2 or more points on the CAGE questionnaire. Alternatively, the AUDIT-C (Bradley et al. 2003; Bush et al. 1998; Table 4–3) is a quick 3-question screen that can reliably identify dangerous alcohol use in adults.

THE SMAST

The Short Michigan Alcoholism Screening Test (SMAST; Selzer et al. 1975) is a more in-depth, 13-question tool to identify adult patients who will require further workup for alcohol abuse (Table 4–4).

Once there is a high suspicion for alcohol misuse, further questions include age at first use, recent patterns of use, and any complications the patient identifies related to use.

On examination, there are many physical stigmata that may raise suspicion for problematic drinking:

- Hepatomegaly
- Splenomegaly
- Spider angiomata
- Gynecomastia
- Testicular atrophy
- Jaundice
- Palmar erythema
- Dupuytren contracture

Several common laboratory abnormalities also are found in those with chronic, heavy alcohol consumption:

- Elevated transaminase levels (classic aspartate transaminase–to–alanine transaminase elevation ratio in alcohol use disorder is 2:1)

TABLE 4–3. Alcohol Use Disorders Identification Test (AUDIT-C) screening tool for problem drinking

1. How often in the past year did you have a drink containing alcohol?

   Never (0—end survey)

   Monthly or less (1)

   2–4× monthly (2)

   2–3× weekly (3)

   4+× weekly (4)

2. How many drinks did you have on a typical day when you were drinking in the past year?

   1 or 2 (0)

   3 or 4 (1)

   5 or 6 (2)

   7–9 (3)

   10+ (4)

3. How often did you have 6 or more drinks on one occasion in the past year?

   Never (0)

   Less than monthly (1)

   Monthly (2)

   Weekly (3)

   Daily or almost daily (4)

A score of 4 or more points is considered positive for males.
A score of 3 or more points is considered positive for females.

Note. Scores are indicated in parentheses after each response.
Source. Bradley et al. 2003; Bush et al. 1998.

TABLE 4–4. Short Michigan Alcoholism Screening Test (SMAST) and scoring for problem drinking severity

These questions refer to the past 12 months only.
Yes=1 point; No=0 points

1. Do you feel that you are a normal drinker? (By *normal,* we mean do you drink less than or as much as most other people?)

2. Does your wife, husband, a parent, or other near relative ever worry or complain about your drinking?

3. Do you ever feel guilty about your drinking?

4. Do friends or relatives think you are a normal drinker?

5. Are you able to stop drinking when you want to?

6. Have you ever attended a meeting of Alcoholics Anonymous (AA)?

7. Has your drinking ever created problems between you and your wife, husband, a parent, or other near relative?

8. Have you ever gotten into trouble at work because of your drinking?

9. Have you ever neglected your obligations, your family, or your work for 2 or more days in a row because you were drinking?

10. Have you ever gone to anyone for help about your drinking?

11. Have you ever been in a hospital because of drinking?

12. Have you ever been arrested for drunken driving, driving while intoxicated, or driving under the influence of alcoholic beverages?

13. Have you ever been arrested, even for a few hours, because of other drunken behaviors?

TABLE 4–4. Short Michigan Alcoholism Screening
Test (SMAST) and scoring for problem
drinking severity *(continued)*

Scoring

0–2: No problems reported; no action needed at this time.

3: Borderline use; further investigation is required.

*4 or more: Potential alcohol use disorder; a full assessment is
required.*

Source. Selzer et al. 1975.

- Hypomagnesemia
- Vitamin deficiencies, such as B_{12} and thiamine
- Macrocytic anemia
- Neutropenia
- Thrombocytopenia
- Increased international normalized ratio

What to Do About Addiction

Approach to treatment depends on the level of severity of the
disease and the patient's goals. For those patients who may
be drinking problematically but do not meet the full criteria
for an alcohol use disorder or meet the criteria for mild alcohol use disorder only, a brief intervention may be used to educate the patient about the potential risks of the drinking
behavior and offer suggestions as to how to moderate or abstain from drinking. Because of the pervasive presence of alcohol consumption in numerous settings, it is not uncommon
for patients to be hesitant about total abstinence. In the spirit
of motivational interviewing (see Chapter 17, "Motivational
Interviewing"), it is best not to challenge this notion but meet
the patient where she or he is in terms of readiness to change
and progress from there.

If a patient with alcohol use disorder has experienced
withdrawal in the past, medically managed withdrawal may
be necessary before further treatment is possible. Please refer
to the section "What to Do About Withdrawal" earlier in this
chapter.

MEDICATIONS

Following detoxification, many patients can benefit from on-going treatment in recovery. Three medications are approved by the U.S. Food and Drug Administration for use in treatment of alcohol use disorder (Center for Substance Abuse Treatment 2009; Saitz and O'Malley 1997).

DISULFIRAM

Disulfiram was the first of the medications for alcohol use disorder and is an irreversible inhibitor of aldehyde dehydrogenase. If a patient taking disulfiram ingests alcohol, this inhibition leads to a buildup of the toxic metabolite acetaldehyde, which produces several unpleasant effects: flushing, sweats, nausea and vomiting, palpitations, and shortness of breath; this is sometimes referred to as a "disulfiram reaction." The reaction occurs within 15 minutes of the ingestion of alcohol. Patients will abstain from alcohol to avoid this aversive stimulus; however, some patients choose to "drink through" the reaction because they will still experience intoxication. Another shortcoming of disulfiram is that patients can decide to simply discontinue the medication and may resume drinking within 2–3 days without triggering the reaction. Thus, disulfiram is often used in structured recovery, when daily directly observed therapy is possible.

Disulfiram can be hepatotoxic, and mild elevation of serum aminotransferase levels occurs in 25% of patients. Overall, the estimated incidence of liver injury is 1 per 10,000–20,000 patient-years. Although quite rare, cases of fulminant hepatic failure have been reported. This dose-independent effect has a mean onset at around 2 months after the initiation of therapy. Unfortunately, this effect develops very rapidly, and no recommended monitoring schedule is guaranteed to detect it; in clinical practice, most practitioners will check liver enzymes monthly for the first 3–6 months and then every 6–12 months thereafter. Disulfiram is usually dosed at 500 mg/day orally for 2 weeks, then the dose is decreased to 250 mg/day orally. In some instances, higher doses may be necessary to provide complete enzyme inhibition. Patients should be abstinent from alcohol for at least 48 hours before starting disulfiram.

NALTREXONE

Naltrexone is a μ opioid antagonist that also has efficacy in reducing opioid use. When used for alcohol use disorder, it is thought to reduce cravings and the rewarding effects of alcohol. Numerous studies have shown an increase in time to relapse and a decrease in the severity of relapse in patients taking naltrexone (Anton et al. 2006; Jonas et al. 2014; Morris et al. 2001; O'Malley et al. 1992). Naltrexone comes in two forms: oral and a once-a-month intramuscular depot injection; dosing for the oral form is 50 mg/day and for the intramuscular form is 380 mg monthly. Depot injection may be preferable for patients for whom compliance is a concern. Naltrexone can be started even in patients who are still actively drinking and in fact may help curb the amount consumed. Gastrointestinal side effects are most common, but other side effects include headache, anxiety, and insomnia.

Naltrexone also can be hepatotoxic, and baseline liver enzymes should be determined before initiation. Naltrexone should not be started if liver enzymes are elevated more than three to five times the upper limit of normal. After initiation, monitoring follows much the same guidelines as for disulfiram, but naltrexone is unlikely to cause fulminant liver failure. Naltrexone should not be started in patients who need chronic opioid treatment for any reason (chronic pain, maintenance therapy for opioid use disorder) because it will block the effects of opioids and cause the patient to experience opioid withdrawal. If a patient taking naltrexone has a known need for a short course of opioids (e.g., after a planned surgery for pain control), naltrexone may be stopped 2–3 days before the procedure and then resumed after the need for opioids has passed.

ACAMPROSATE

Acamprosate has a structure similar to taurine. Although its exact mechanism of action is unknown, it is thought to modulate and/or inhibit glutamate receptors, which may reduce negative reinforcement under alcohol deprivation. Like naltrexone, acamprosate reduces drinking by reducing alcohol craving. Acamprosate is dosed at 333 mg or 666 mg orally three times a day and is initiated after the patient has already stopped drinking for a brief period (it is often started during detoxification). The most common side effects are nausea and headache. Acamprosate may be a good choice for patients with significantly impaired liver function because it is renally excreted.

PSYCHOSOCIAL TREATMENTS

For most individuals, psychosocial treatments will be necessary in addition to medication in order to recover from an alcohol use disorder. These interventions can occur in many different settings, and many different modalities of therapy have been shown to be of benefit to this patient population. These are covered in later chapters (see Part III, "Treatment").

ALCOHOLICS ANONYMOUS

One particular tool that is an important part of recovery for many people with alcohol use disorder is Alcoholics Anonymous (AA). Founded in 1935, AA is an international, peer-support fellowship of people who have had difficulty with alcohol use. It is a self-sustaining nonprofessional organization and has no requirements for membership other than an individual's desire to tackle his or her drinking problem (Alcoholics Anonymous 2001). The most well-known facet of this program is the Twelve Steps (discussed further in Chapter 18, "Twelve-Step Programs and Spirituality"), which participants must "work" in order to progress on their path to recovery. Many other "Anonymous" programs have come into existence over the years (e.g., Narcotics Anonymous, Crystal Meth Anonymous, Overeaters Anonymous), all of which are based on this original model.

AA has helped many individuals find sobriety over the decades and can be a very helpful part of a patient's treatment regimen, but it is not the only way to recovery. One facet of AA to which some patients object is the emphasis on spirituality, and other peer-support groups such as Self-Management and Recovery Training (SMART) or Rational Recovery do not have this same focus and may be more appealing.

Special Issues With Psychiatric Comorbidities

Co-occurring psychiatric disorders are very common in patients with alcohol use disorder; mood disorders (major depressive disorder, bipolar disorder), anxiety disorders (generalized anxiety disorder and social phobia), and post-traumatic stress disorder are among the most commonly diagnosed. Those patients with both alcohol use disorder and another psychiatric disorder tend to have a more severe and difficult-to-treat course than do patients with only a single diagnosis. Untreated psychiatric symptoms can lead to worsening substance abuse, refractoriness to treatment, and increased risk for suicide. Thus, it is important in initial assessment to screen for other psychiatric disorders and to treat them in conjunction with addiction treatment.

One of the more challenging tasks for the clinician is to determine whether psychiatric symptoms are due to an underlying psychiatric co-occurring illness or are substance-induced. A careful history is a crucial first step toward unraveling this conundrum. Asking about the temporal relation between the initiation of substance use and the development of psychiatric symptoms can help to start to clarify this issue, as can asking about any psychiatric symptoms during the patient's periods of sobriety. As the relationship with the patient develops over time, there will be further opportunity to observe and learn about the interplay between alcohol use and psychiatric symptoms. In some settings such as the correctional system, 28-day rehabilitation programs, or long-term residential programs, there may be the opportunity to directly observe the patient in an environment where abstinence is nearly ensured.

Special Issues With Medical Comorbidities

Alcohol has a multitude of negative effects across myriad organ systems and can cause end-organ damage with chronic, heavy use. The toxic effects of alcohol on the liver are well known and range from mild transaminitis (which can occur after even one episode of heavy drinking) to end-stage liver disease. Between 10% and 20% of heavy drinkers will develop cirrhosis. Many other medical problems can develop, and the following are only a sampling.

- Gastrointestinal: Mallory-Weiss tears, Boerhaave syndrome, varices, gastritis, and increased risk for gastric carcinoma
- Cardiovascular: cardiomyopathy, hypertension, and "holiday heart"
- Musculoskeletal: decreased bone mass
- CNS: decreased neuronal volume in the anterior hippocampus; damage to mammillary bodies (Korsakoff syndrome), corpus callosum (Marchiafava-Bignami disease), and frontal lobes

Patients can present with multiple medical comorbidities related to alcohol use disorder and are often best managed with a cooperative, multidisciplinary team.

Special Issues With Specific Populations: Pregnancy

Alcohol is a teratogen, and multiple professional entities such as the Centers for Disease Control and Prevention, U.S. Surgeon General, American Congress of Obstetrics and Gynecology, and American Academy of Pediatrics have issued statements that no safe amount or kind of alcohol can be consumed during pregnancy, and no time during pregnancy is safe for drinking. Alcohol crosses the placental barrier easily and can stunt fetal growth and damage developing CNS structures, as well as cause several recognizable physical changes. Fetal alcohol exposure is the leading preventable cause of intellectual disability in the United States. Women who are pregnant should be counseled about alcohol consumption, and further specialized treatment for alcohol use disorder should be available as well.

KEY POINTS

Alcohol is one of the oldest, most pervasively used and misused psychoactive substances in the world. Despite its legal status and social acceptability in many countries, it remains a potentially dangerous, toxic substance with significant individual and social effects.

Withdrawal from alcohol can be fatal, and medically managed withdrawal is often necessary to ensure safe cessation of alcohol use. Serious syndromes such as withdrawal seizures and delirium tremens require treatment in more intensive settings such as a hospital-based detoxification unit or medical unit.

Three medications are approved by the U.S. Food and Drug Administration for treatment of alcohol use disorder: acamprosate, naltrexone, and disulfiram. Selection of a treatment is dependent on individual circumstance and preference, and these medications also can be used in combination with one another. In addition, psychosocial treatments are an important part of most patients' recovery journeys.

Chronic, heavy alcohol use affects multiple organ systems, and patients frequently have numerous medical and psychiatric comorbidities that require coordinated management along with their substance use treatment to ensure stabilization and recovery.

References

Alcoholics Anonymous: Alcoholics Anonymous, 4th Edition. New York, Alcoholics Anonymous World Services, 2001

American Psychiatric Association: Diagnostic and Statistical Manual of Mental Disorders, 5th Edition. Arlington, VA, American Psychiatric Association, 2013

Anton RF, O'Malley SS, Ciraulo DA, et al: Combined pharmacotherapies and behavioral interventions for alcohol dependence: the COMBINE study: a randomized controlled trial. JAMA 295(17):2003–2017, 2006 16670409

Bradley KA, Bush KR, Epler AJ, et al: Two brief alcohol-screening tests from the Alcohol Use Disorders Identification Test (AUDIT): validation in a female Veterans Affairs patient population. Arch Intern Med 163(7):821–829, 2003 12695273

Bush K, Kivlahan DR, McDonell MB, et al: The AUDIT alcohol consumption questions (AUDIT-C): an effective brief screening test for problem drinking. Ambulatory Care Quality Improvement Project (ACQUIP). Alcohol Use Disorders Identification Test. Arch Intern Med 158(16):1789–1795, 1998 9738608

Center for Substance Abuse Treatment: Incorporating Alcohol Pharmacotherapies Into Medical Practice (Treatment Improvement Protocol [TIP] series, 49). Rockville, MD, Substance Abuse and Mental Health Services Administration, 2009

Centers for Disease Control and Prevention: Excessive Drinking Costs U.S. $223.5 Billion. April 17, 2014. Available at: http://www.cdc.gov/features/alcoholconsumption. Accessed December 11, 2015.

Greenfield LA: Alcohol and Crime: An Analysis of National Data on the Prevalence of Alcohol Involvement in Crime Washington, DC, U.S. Department of Justice, Bureau of Justice Statistics, 1998. Available at: http://www.bjs.gov/content/pub/pdf/ac.pdf. Accessed February 24, 2016.

Hasin DS, Stinson FS, Ogburn E, Grant BF: Prevalence, correlates, disability, and comorbidity of DSM-IV alcohol abuse and dependence in the United States: results from the National Epidemiologic Survey on Alcohol and Related Conditions. Arch Gen Psychiatry 64(7):830–842, 2007 17606817

Jonas DE, Amick HR, Feltner C, et al: Pharmacotherapy for adults with alcohol use disorders in outpatient settings: a systematic review and meta-analysis. JAMA 311(18):1889–1900, 2014 24825644

Morris PL, Hopwood M, Whelan G, et al: Naltrexone for alcohol dependence: a randomized controlled trial. Addiction 96(11):1565–1573, 2001 11784454

National Institute on Alcohol Abuse and Alcoholism: Alcohol Use and Alcohol Use Disorders in the United States, A 3-Year Follow-Up: Main Findings From the 2004–2005 Wave 2 National Epidemiologic Survey on Alcohol and Related Conditions (NESARC). Bethesda, MD, National Institutes of Health, 2010. Available at: http://pubs.niaaa.nih.gov/publications/NESARC_DRM2/NESARC2DRM.pdf. Accessed December 11, 2015.

O'Malley SS, Jaffe AJ, Chang G, et al: Naltrexone and coping skills therapy for alcohol dependence: a controlled study. Arch Gen Psychiatry 49(11):881–887, 1992 1444726

Saitz R, O'Malley SS: Pharmacotherapies for alcohol abuse: withdrawal and treatment. Med Clin North Am 81(4):881–907, 1997 9222259

Selzer ML, Vinokur A, van Rooijen L: A self-administered Short Michigan Alcoholism Screening Test (SMAST). J Stud Alcohol 36(1):117–126, 1975 238068

Sullivan JT, Sykora K, Schneiderman J, et al: Assessment of alcohol withdrawal: the revised clinical institute withdrawal assessment for alcohol scale (CIWA-Ar). Br J Addict 84(11):1353–1357, 1989 2597811

CHAPTER 5

Anabolic-Androgenic Steroids

CHERYL A. KENNEDY, M.D.

TSHERING BHUTIA, M.B.B.S.

ANABOLIC-androgenic steroids have both androgenic (masculinizing) and anabolic (muscle-building) effects. Anabolic-androgenic steroids are also called appearance- and performance-enhancing drugs. These substances are all synthetic derivatives of testosterone, are widely sought after, and are easily obtained through a huge international illicit trade and, more locally, through gyms and some trainers and physicians. Because these drugs are created in a laboratory (not plant based), their routes of synthesis and distribution originate from constantly evolving and innovative sources. All testosterone-like compounds and a large variety of other substances (diuretics, blood-forming stimulants, other agents used to "dope") are banned in sports inside and outside competition. An international independent agency established in 1999 and composed of and funded equally by the sports movement and world governments, the World Anti-Doping Agency (2015) regularly updates the banned substances list.

Used medically, certain anabolic-androgenic steroids that are approved by the U.S. Food and Drug Administration are controlled substances on Drug Enforcement Administration Schedule III, defining them as substances with medical uses that may cause low to moderate physical dependence or high psychological dependence. Anabolic-androgenic steroids are used medically for a variety of conditions:

- Growth stimulation in children at low growth percentiles (being replaced by human growth hormone)
- Induction of delayed male puberty

- Appetite stimulation, muscle mass preservation in wasting conditions: cancer, AIDS
- Bone marrow stimulation (being replaced by epoetin alfa, which directly stimulates blood cell precursors)
- Male hormone replacement in those with low levels
- Gender reassignment for various conditions
- Increase of libido in older men

The updated Designer Anabolic Steroid Control Act of 2014 (P.L. 113-260) broadened the definition of anabolic steroids to include all related "designer" substances that originate from synthetic testosterone-like compounds. This effectively includes all current and future compounds, but enforcement and interdiction have proved difficult given the easy availability of these substances through Internet providers and other illicit means. Since the perceived positive effects of anabolic-androgenic steroids have become known, chemical variations continuously are available, and they are easy to obtain outside standard medical practice. Because of the steroid use scandals throughout professional sports (e.g., cycling, baseball, football, swimming, track and field) since the 1990s, elite athletes are not currently the main anabolic-androgenic steroid users, but rather adolescent boys and young adult males, most of whom are not athletes. Athletes have not abandoned "doping" to gain a competitive edge, but there is a constant search to evade detection, and users often are willing to try other types of drugs as well.

Pharmacology

Anabolic-androgenic steroids can affect many body parts and tissues, including skin, muscle, bone, liver, and kidneys, as well as hematopoietic, immune, reproductive, and central nervous systems (Barceloux and Palmer 2013). Rapidly evolving with many analogues and derivatives, anabolic-androgenic steroid pharmacology is poorly studied, and some mechanisms of action and effective dosing to achieve specific outcomes are not known. During fetal development, endogenous anabolic-androgenic steroids exert growth on internal and external genitalia. In an effort to create different anabolic-androgenic effect ratios or change absorption affinities, pharmacologists use three major chemical techniques (Joseph and Parr 2015):

1. Alkylation at the 17-α position with an ethyl or a methyl group produces orally absorbed compounds with slowed hepatic metabolism.
2. Esterification at the 17-β position creates a compound that can be parenterally administered and has a prolonged mechanism of action as a result of lipid solubility.
3. Alterations in the ring structure of both parenteral and oral compounds alter the anabolic-androgenic ratios, producing differential effects.

Receptor studies are rapidly expanding the pharmacological complexities of these compounds.

During normal puberty, increased androgenic steroid production in the testes fosters

- Further growth of external genitalia
- Growth of male accessory reproductive glands (prostate, seminal vesicles)
- Secretory activity

Androgenic enhancement of secondary sexual characteristics of puberty produces

- Larynx enlargement with deepening voice
- Terminal hair growth (pubic, axillary, facial)
- Sebaceous gland activity (can lead to acne)
- Central nervous system effects (increased libido and aggression)

Anabolic effects during puberty include

- Growth of muscle and bone
- End of linear bone growth with epiphysis closure

Anabolic-androgenic steroids, as fat-soluble molecules, cross cell membrane barriers, bind to androgen receptors centrally and peripherally with varying affinities depending on the compound, and exert direct effects on cell nuclei, altering gene expression or sending a second message to other cell parts. Specific androgenic effects are accomplished through increased protein synthesis that increases appetite and muscular, skeletal, hair, gonadal, and blood cell growth. Effects include growth of clitoris in girls or penis in boys, and, with exogenous administration, suppression of normal sex hormones, impaired sperm production, and increased libido. Females can get unwanted facial hair, loss of breast tissue, and voice deepening. Males develop gynecomastia (breast enlargement), testicular atrophy, and reduced sperm count.

Most nonmedical users reach supraphysiological doses, and depending on length of use, some effects may be irreversible. These substances are hormones, and disproportionate use can disrupt normal endocrine function and lead to long-term adverse effects. Anabolic-androgenic steroids also interfere with the metabolism of other therapeutics such as cyclosporine and warfarin, resulting in dangerously higher drug levels.

Anabolic-androgenic steroids are administered through various routes:

- Oral: most convenient; the small absorbable fraction is difficult for the liver to metabolize completely and may be responsible for adverse long-term effects. (Table 5–1 lists common oral anabolic-androgenic steroids.)
- Injectable forms: most common form of use; mainly intramuscular; if intravenous, lipid solubility can cause embolism or rapid changes in hormone levels. (Table 5–2 lists common injectable anabolic-androgenic steroids.)
- Topical preparations, including the following:
  - Topical creams, gels, lotions, and ointments
  - Sprays and solutions
  - Transdermal patches

With all anabolic-androgenic steroid preparations, but especially topical preparations (as noted above), precautions must be taken with women and children. This population is extremely susceptible to dramatic, dangerous, and adverse effects from even very tiny amounts easily and accidentally absorbed through the skin.

Toxicology

Detecting anabolic-androgenic steroid use has bedeviled organized sports for decades, and toxicological analysis remains complex and is not routine in health care settings. No reliable "point of care" testing is available because sophisticated laboratory methods are needed to reliably detect and

TABLE 5–1. Common oral anabolic-androgenic steroids

Generic name	Trade name	Street name
Oxymetholone	Anadrol	Drol
Testosterone undecanoate	Andriol	Andy
Metenolone	Primobolan	Primo
Oxandrolone	Anavar	Var
Stanozolol	Winstrol	Winny
Fluoxymesterone	Halotestin	Halo
4-Chlorodehydromethyl-testosterone	Turinabol	Tbol

Note. Trade and street names may vary and change over time.

TABLE 5–2. Common injectable anabolic-androgenic steroids, including longer-acting "depot" preparations (decanoates)

Generic name	Trade name	Street name
Nandrolone decanoate	Deca-Durabolin	Deca
Boldenone undecylenate	Equipoise	EQ
Drostanolone propionate	Masteron	Only referred to by trade name
Nandrolone phenylpropionate	Various	NPP
Methenolone enanthate	Primobolan Depot	Primo
Trenbolone	No common trade name	Tren
Testosterone	Various	Test
Stanozolol depot	Winstrol Depot	Winny

Note. Trade and street names may vary and change over time.

identify the varied compounds and many metabolites. Workplace and sensitive worker testing does not usually include anabolic-androgenic steroids but rather these five substances or metabolites: amphetamines, cocaine, cannabis, opioids, and phencyclidine.

Specialized assay techniques are used to differentiate endogenous (made in the body) hormones from exogenous (made outside the body) sources. It is agreed that rapid ultrahigh performance liquid chromatography tandem mass spectrometry has become the technique of choice for anabolic steroid analysis. Detection time from last dose varies from a few days to weeks and months depending on the compound, amount used, and method of use. Some users also abuse diuretics and other drugs and use fluid manipulation techniques to increase urine flow and sodium excretion, adjust volume and composition of body fluids, and chemically change assays in an attempt to mask and complicate detection (Cadwallader et al. 2010).

How to Recognize Use

Various methods and regimens are used to take anabolic-androgenic steroids. These include mixing, cycling, stacking, and pyramiding. Users often take more than one compound or whatever anabolic-androgenic steroid they can obtain. Sources providing steroids are not always honest, and users can get weak compounds or completely inactive drugs. Users often take increasing doses over time: cycling or stacking one compound on top of another in a cycle; other users may pyramid their use by gradually titrating doses upward and then gradually tapering doses downward. Compounding cycles over weeks or months and escalating doses lead to supraphysiological levels that induce dramatic and adverse effects.

Anabolic-androgenic steroids remain unusual among drugs of abuse because the usual markers of impairment or euphoria are not obvious or typically associated with illicit drug use. Rather, anabolic-androgenic steroids seem to lower the threshold for a constellation of behaviors that span irritability, anger, frank rage, and mania spiked with aggression ("roid rage"). Users often have a cluster of rewarding or impulsive behaviors that include aggression, hypersexual behavior, and strict dietary regimens with supplements, often including diuretics, exercise, and other drug use. Most users are adolescents and young adult males, heterosexual or gay, who are either amateur athletes or involved in weight lifting and the bodybuilding culture; and, although use among elite athletes is lower, the use of these agents nonetheless remains in this population. Studies indicate that anabolic-androgenic steroid users do not trust physicians and fail to disclose use; most physicians do not inquire about these drugs. Users research drugs on their own through peer groups in gyms and through Internet sources (Kanayama et al. 2010).

Clinicians should obtain a detailed medical, psychiatric, and drug use history and perform a comprehensive physical examination, keeping the following list in mind. Care must be taken with heavily tattooed skin to be thorough. Clinicians should collect collateral information from family, friends, or medical records. The following are some signs that suggest anabolic-androgenic steroid use and essential endocrine disruption:

- Behavior or mood changes: irritability, aggression, mood swings, mania, increased sexual activity, frank paranoia, isolation from others, suicidal depression, especially in withdrawal
- Peripheral puncture marks or skin infections (injection drug use)
- Small testis
- Enlarged prostate
- Small red or purple acne patches, especially on upper back and shoulders
- Gynecomastia
- Extra-greasy or oily hair
- Cutaneous striae, especially in deltoid and pectoral areas
- Use of other drugs or alcohol
- Elevated blood pressure
- Obsessional focus on exercise, bodybuilding, diet, and dietary supplements
- Evidence of body dysmorphic disorder
- In female athletes, bodybuilders, assault survivors: hirsutism, balding, acne, and menstrual disruption

Laboratory values:

- Elevated glucose level
- Decreased high-density lipoprotein level

- Increased low-density lipoprotein level
- Abnormal liver function test results

Muscle dysmorphic disorder may be a subtype of body dysmorphic disorder. Like those with eating disorders, these individuals are obsessed with appearance but think they are skinny and puny when they are actually strong and muscular looking. They disguise their bodies with loose-fitting clothing and are insecure about their appearance or exposing their bodies. They pay excessive and inordinate attention to diet, supplements, and workouts so that it often interferes with other activities or duties (Substance Abuse and Mental Health Services Administration 2006).

TOLERANCE

Tolerance is a minimally researched, poorly understood concept in regard to anabolic-androgenic steroids. Anabolic-androgenic steroids are difficult to measure; users often follow very individualized patterns of use, with the tendency to sequence different substances in varying amounts. Drug potency varies widely, and few clinical pharmacological data are available on many anabolic-androgenic steroids. Many users do not even know what they are taking or, worse, are taking a different drug from what they thought. Blood levels vary greatly given the variety of compounds and characteristics. If tolerance is applied to anabolic-androgenic steroid use, it occurs when large doses or longer duration of anabolic-androgenic steroid use no longer produces the desired effect. This effect might be changes in muscle mass or in general appearance, but users may uniquely distort this determination, particularly those with body dysmorphic disorder or another psychiatric condition that drives use (Pagonis et al. 2006).

DSM-5 criteria for other (or unknown) substance use disorder (Box 5–1; American Psychiatric Association 2013) are applicable for the diagnosis of anabolic-androgenic steroid use disorder.

Box 5–1.   Diagnostic Criteria for Other (or Unknown)
                 Substance Use Disorder

A. A problematic pattern of use of an intoxicating substance not able to be classified within the alcohol; caffeine; cannabis; hallucinogen (phencyclidine and others); inhalant; opioid; sedative, hypnotic, or anxiolytic; stimulant; or tobacco categories and leading to clinically significant impairment or distress, as manifested by at least two of the following, occurring within a 12-month period:

1. The substance is often taken in larger amounts or over a longer period than was intended.
2. There is a persistent desire or unsuccessful efforts to cut down or control use of the substance.
3. A great deal of time is spent in activities necessary to obtain the substance, use the substance, or recover from its effects.
4. Craving, or a strong desire or urge to use the substance.
5. Recurrent use of the substance resulting in a failure to fulfill major role obligations at work, school, or home.
6. Continued use of the substance despite having persistent or recurrent social or interpersonal problems caused or exacerbated by the effects of its use.
7. Important social, occupational, or recreational activities are given up or reduced because of use of the substance.
8. Recurrent use of the substance in situations in which it is physically hazardous.
9. Use of the substance is continued despite knowledge of having a persistent or recurrent physical or psychological problem that is likely to have been caused or exacerbated by the substance.
10. Tolerance, as defined by either of the following:
    a. A need for markedly increased amounts of the substance to achieve intoxication or desired effect.
    b. A markedly diminished effect with continued use of the same amount of the substance.
11. Withdrawal, as manifested by either of the following:
    a. The characteristic withdrawal syndrome for other (or unknown) substance (refer to Criteria A and B of the criteria sets for other [or unknown] substance withdrawal).
    b. The substance (or a closely related substance) is taken to relieve or avoid withdrawal symptoms.

Specify if:
In early remission

In sustained remission

Specify if:
In a controlled environment

Specify current severity:
Mild: Presence of 2–3 symptoms.
Moderate: Presence of 4–5 symptoms.
Severe: Presence of 6 or more symptoms.

- Hepatitis A, B, and C and HIV
- Liver dysfunction, cholestatic jaundice, hepatic tumors, and hepatic and/or splenic peliosis (focal liver necrosis and fibrosis)
- Cardiomyopathy, atherosclerotic disease, valve disease, atrial fibrillation, stroke, myocardial infarction, dyslipidemia, hypertension, and thrombotic events
- Mood instability, morbid depression with ongoing suicide risk, and anxiety
- Sometimes irreversible: testicular atrophy, enlarged clitoris, abnormal hair distribution, hirsutism, gynecomastia, infertility, voice depth, and short stature in adolescents

The anabolic-androgenic steroid genomic actions that promote hormonal and protein syntheses may be the initial provocation for starting use (i.e., for enhanced appearance or strength), but for some, pathological dysmorphia, dysphoria, or hypogonadism is the impetus for continued use and ongoing dependence and addiction. Long-term dependence engenders addiction behaviors like those seen with other drugs of abuse. Those who use anabolic-androgenic steroids, especially chronically, are also at higher risk for using other drugs, particularly opioids and stimulants, than are those who do not use steroids (Pope et al. 2014).

What to Do About Intoxication

Anabolic-androgenic steroids are not generally thought to cause acute intoxication like other "hedonic" drugs. Users do not, initially, take these drugs to obtain the classic drug high, but anabolic-androgenic steroids are psychotropic and have physiological reinforcing effects that increase feelings of self-confidence and aggressiveness.

Acute toxicity is rare, but users can develop acute gastrointestinal upset that can be treated with calcium- or magnesium-based antacids, proton pump inhibitors, or H_2 blockers. Other types of acute complications from injecting (e.g., endocarditis, cellulitis) or hypersensitivity reactions should be managed appropriately.

A wide range of psychiatric symptoms can be induced by anabolic-androgenic steroid use. Some users report mania, hypomania, irritability, anger, and poor impulse control. These can be acute and dangerous and should be treated as emergencies. The intensity of effects and variety of symptoms increase as use increases. More prolonged and high-dose use increases the risk for long-term complications. Many myths about anabolic-androgenic steroids make them appear to be low risk, particularly for impressionable or vulnerable youths or those with a psychological need to be big and strong, including some athletes, insecure teenagers, young adult males (mainly), and assault survivors. Some myths include the erroneous beliefs that anabolic-androgenic steroids are "not harmful," are "not as addictive" or "not as illegal" as some other drugs, or "don't really stunt growth" and that "all steroids are pretty much the same." Anabolic-androgenic steroids, because of their hormonal nature, can and do have the additional biological effects of major endocrine disruption.

DSM-5 criteria for other (or unknown) substance intoxication (Box 5–2) are applicable for the diagnosis of anabolic-androgenic steroid intoxication.

Box 5–2.   Diagnostic Criteria for Other (or Unknown) Substance Intoxication

---

A. The development of a reversible substance-specific syndrome attributable to recent ingestion of (or exposure to) a substance that is not listed elsewhere or is unknown.

B. Clinically significant problematic behavioral or psychological changes that are attributable to the effect of the substance on the central nervous system (e.g., impaired motor coordination, psychomotor agitation or retardation, euphoria, anxiety, belligerence, mood lability, cognitive impairment, impaired judgment, social withdrawal) and develop during, or shortly after, use of the substance.

C. The signs or symptoms are not attributable to another medical condition and are not better explained by another mental disorder, including intoxication with another substance.

How to Recognize Withdrawal

Some users, especially with prolonged use and high (supraphysiological) doses, may have suppression of the hypothalamic-pituitary-gonadal axis and hypogonadism. This effect can persist long after anabolic-androgenic steroid use is discontinued. The primary effects of hypogonadism and other neuroendocrine factors lead to a well-characterized anabolic-androgenic steroid withdrawal syndrome with

- Dysphoric "craving"
- Decreased libido
- Classic flu-like syndrome with fatigue, joint and muscle pain, headache, and insomnia
- Depression and suicidal ideation
- Decreased stamina
- Decreased exercise tolerance
- Diminished muscle tone and contour

DSM-5 criteria for other (or unknown) substance withdrawal (Box 5–3) are applicable for the diagnosis of anabolic-androgenic steroid withdrawal.

Box 5–3. Diagnostic Criteria for Other (or Unknown) Substance Withdrawal

---

A. Cessation of (or reduction in) use of a substance that has been heavy and prolonged.

B. The development of a substance-specific syndrome shortly after the cessation of (or reduction in) substance use.

C. The substance-specific syndrome causes clinically significant distress or impairment in social, occupational, or other important areas of functioning.

D. The symptoms are not attributable to another medical condition and are not better explained by another mental disorder, including withdrawal from another substance.

E. The substance involved cannot be classified under any of the other substance categories (alcohol; caffeine; cannabis; opioids; sedatives, hypnotics, or anxiolytics; stimulants; or tobacco) or is unknown.

Patients getting therapeutic hormone replacement for testicular failure may be more emotionally labile with mood swings just before dosage due date for hormone replacement. This can be addressed by administration of lower doses of testosterone enanthate divided throughout the month or continuous administration with patches or gels that eliminate big variations in blood levels (Hochberg et al. 2003).

Treatment

Most anabolic-androgenic steroid users do not present for treatment. Long-term users who started in the 1980s and 1990s are reaching the age of risk for the well-documented cardiac and psychoneuroendocrine complications of long-term anabolic-androgenic steroid use. This may motivate some to seek treatment. The acute flu-like syndrome seen in withdrawal has been ameliorated by administration of clonidine, tranquilizers, and analgesics. Therapeutic effects have been reported from use of the antidepressant fluoxetine or other selective serotonin reuptake inhibitors (SSRIs) in treating the androgen withdrawal syndrome. Naltrexone has been tried with some success.

Another approach might be hormone substitution or replacement therapy and very gradual dose tapering (differing opinions). Some practitioners have used chorionic gonadotropin treatment or clomiphene to stimulate the neuroendocrine system. This is indicated only with a reliable patient committed to termination of anabolic-androgenic steroid use with clinical hypogonadism that warrants replacement therapy until recovery of the hypothalamic-pituitary-gonadal axis.

Addicted anabolic-androgenic steroid users can benefit from strategies and techniques used with classic drugs of abuse, particularly individuals with long-term use and classic addiction behaviors (see Part III, "Treatment"). Individuals with disturbance in body image with body dysmorphic disorder may benefit from SSRIs and cognitive-behavioral therapy designed to reduce compulsive behaviors. A sports-minded nutritionist and physical trainer can develop healthy methods to make and maintain muscle strength and desirable body image without anabolic-androgenic steroids (Kanayama et al. 2010).

Special Issues With Psychiatric and Medical Comorbidities

Much like the challenge posed by treating addiction in patients with HIV, hepatitis C virus, or cirrhosis, persons addicted to anabolic-androgenic steroids need case management and a strongly integrated multidisciplinary and interprofessional team in a patient-centered care environment. Culturally well-versed mental health and other substance use disorders counselors ideally would be well integrated to maximize effectiveness of all treatments. Multiple serious medical comorbidities are stressful for patients and providers. Health beliefs, culture, socioeconomic status, and ethnicity will affect outcomes. Anabolic-androgenic steroid users have varied and disparate cultures, and each poses its own difficulties in treatment.

Special Issues With Specific Populations

Among certain groups in the bodybuilding culture (both gay and heterosexual) and among some athletes, the risk of using anabolic-androgenic steroids, aside from the illegality, is underappreciated and minimized. Some younger users—often, susceptible adolescents or those being mentored by more successful athletes, bodybuilders, or unscrupulous coaches—do not understand the risks they are taking. The culture supports networks of users and those who transmit "knowledge" and state that the "benefit outweighs the risk." Many users do not trust physicians and take what is offered from other users as valid. Anabolic-androgenic steroids are sold on various Web sites (they are legal in some countries), chat forums are used to exchange information, some Web sites are dedicated to sharing methods designed to avoid detection, and others purport to provide "valid" information. Legitimate health and safety sites have accurate medical information. Research is minimal because of the variety of these substances, lack of standardization in use, expense and difficulty of detection methods, and ethical issues in human research. Primary prevention education programs within the health education curricula of school-age youths could provide all students with accurate and medically relevant information.

Harm reduction is a secondary prevention strategy for those not ready to stop using. Use of clean, sterile needles and hepatitis vaccines, along with continued motivational counseling and health education to support abstinence, are indicated.

KEY POINTS

Anabolic-androgenic steroids comprise numerous basic and designer compounds that are difficult to detect.

Widespread "underground trade," mainly via the Internet, complicates interdiction and enforcement.

Adolescents and young adult males are at highest risk for anabolic-androgenic steroid use.

Short- and long-term use of anabolic-androgenic steroids increases risk for adverse outcomes.

Psychiatric conditions can be both a source for the drive to use and an adverse outcome of anabolic-androgenic steroid use.

References

American Psychiatric Association: Diagnostic and Statistical Manual of Mental Disorders, 5th Edition. Arlington, VA, American Psychiatric Association, 2013

Barceloux DG, Palmer RB: Anabolic-androgenic steroids. Dis Mon 59(6):226–248, 2013 23719201

Cadwallader AB, de la Torre X, Tieri A, Botrè F: The abuse of diuretics as performance-enhancing drugs and masking agents in sport doping: pharmacology, toxicology and analysis. Br J Pharmacol 161(1):1–16, 2010 20718736

Designer Anabolic Steroid Control Act of 2014, Pub. L. No. 113-260, December 18, 2014. Available at: https://www.congress.gov/bill/113th-congress/house-bill/4771/text. Accessed February 24, 2016.

Hochberg Z, Pacak K, Chrousos GP: Endocrine withdrawal syndromes. Endocr Rev 24(4):523–538, 2003 12920153

Joseph JF, Parr MK: Synthetic androgens as designer supplements. Curr Neuropharmacol 13(1):89–100, 2015 26074745

Kanayama G, Brower KJ, Wood RI, et al: Treatment of anabolic-androgenic steroid dependence: emerging evidence and its implications. Drug Alcohol Depend 109(1–3):6–13, 2010 20188494

Pagonis TA, Angelopoulos NV, Koukoulis GN, et al: Psychiatric side effects induced by supraphysiological doses of combinations of anabolic steroids correlate to the severity of abuse. Eur Psychiatry 21(8):551–562, 2006 16356691

Pope HG Jr, Wood RI, Rogol A, et al: Adverse health consequences of performance-enhancing drugs: an Endocrine Society scientific statement. Endocr Rev 35(3):341–375, 2014 24423981

Substance Abuse and Mental Health Services Administration: Anabolic Steroids. Substance Abuse Treatment Advisory, Vol 5, Issue 3. Rockville, MD, Substance Abuse and Mental Health Services Administration, June 2006

World Anti-Doping Agency: Who We Are. 2015. Available at: https://www.wada-ama.org/en/who-we-are. Accessed January 31, 2015.

CHAPTER 6

Benzodiazepines

VICKI KALIRA, M.D.

BENZODIAZEPINES remain some of the most commonly prescribed agents in primary care today. Although they have been used since the 1960s for the management of insomnia and anxiety, with prolonged use, benzodiazepines can contribute to worsening of these symptoms.

Benzodiazepines have been approved by the U.S. Food and Drug Administration for panic disorder, social phobia, generalized anxiety disorder, insomnia, and seizures and as premedication for anesthetic procedures. They are the drugs of choice for the inpatient treatment of alcohol withdrawal, given documented efficacy and safety profiles. All benzodiazepines are effective, but agents without active metabolites, such as lorazepam or oxazepam, are preferred in those with liver impairment.

Efforts have been made to minimize the use of benzodiazepines by using selective serotonin reuptake inhibitors (SSRIs) for anxiety and nonsedative hypnotics for sleep; however, the 2015 Beers Criteria now states the following:

> The nonbenzodiazepine, benzodiazepine receptor agonist hypnotics (eszopiclone, zaleplon, zolpidem) are to be avoided without consideration of duration of use because of their association with harms balanced with their minimal efficacy in treating insomnia. (American Geriatrics Society 2015 Beers Criteria Update Expert Panel 2015, p. 4)

In addition, there remains a general lack of knowledge and understanding of the long-term effects of benzodiazepines. For example, a recent finding indicates that benzodiazepines may lead to early-onset Alzheimer's dementia (Billioti de Gage et al. 2014).

In general, benzodiazepines should be avoided when possible, especially in the elderly and those with current or past substance abuse. Benzodiazepines may be considered as temporary adjuncts but require close monitoring and reassessment of need. Before clinicians prescribe a benzodiazepine, patients should be counseled on lethal interactions, including with alcohol given cross-tolerance and with opioids given central nervous system (CNS) depression. If prescribing, the clinician should first confirm that the patient is not already taking a similar agent by calling the pharmacy or checking the state's controlled substance patient database (e.g., I-STOP in New York). Agents with lower abuse potential are preferred, such as clonazepam as opposed to alprazolam.

Pharmacology

Benzodiazepines potentiate the effect of the inhibitory neurotransmitter γ-aminobutyric acid (GABA) by binding to the $GABA_A$ receptor and producing an allosteric change. This modification causes GABA to bind more tightly, allowing chloride ions into the inhibitory interneuron, leading to hyperpolarization and neuronal inhibition. The net effect is less inhibition on dopaminergic neurons and resultant dopamine release and reinforcement (Olsen and Betz 2006). The $GABA_A$ receptor complex is made up of five subunits. Receptors containing α_1, α_2, α_3, and α_5 subunits are sensitive to the effects of benzodiazepines (see Table 6–1 for additional details).

TABLE 6–1. Benzodiazepine-sensitive γ-aminobutyric acid A ($GABA_A$) receptor subtypes

Type	Action
α_1	Sedative-hypnotic effects, ataxia
α_2, α_3	Antianxiety effects, muscle relaxation
α_5	Sedation, amnesia

Most benzodiazepines undergo oxidative metabolism by cytochrome P450 (CYP) 3A4 first and then glucuronidation. Lorazepam and oxazepam undergo direct glucuronidation and have no active metabolites and are therefore preferred in patients with hepatic impairment.

Benzodiazepines are lipid soluble, allowing for relatively rapid onset of action as well as protracted duration of action with sequestration into body fat; benzodiazepines with active metabolites have an extended effect. Activation of the $GABA_A$ receptor produces sedation, anxiolysis, amnesia, muscle relaxation, and increased seizure threshold. Evidence indicates that anxiety disorders are associated with GABA receptor dysregulation.

Long-term benzodiazepine use leads to tolerance secondary to downregulation of GABA receptors and a compensatory upregulation of the excitatory glutamate system. Rates of tolerance and withdrawal differ per agent; as expected, those with shorter half-lives tend to lead more quickly to tolerance and withdrawal. Benzodiazepines have varying serum half-lives. For a list of commonly used benzodiazepines and their properties (including equivalent doses), see Table 6–2.

Benzodiazepines can be taken by a variety of routes:

- Oral
- Intranasal (recreational use)
- Intravenous injection
- Intramuscular injection
- Rectal
- Smoking (recreational use)

TOXICOLOGY

It is important to determine which metabolite is being assayed in a toxicology screen. Most routine urine immunoassays for benzodiazepines will detect unconjugated oxazepam and therefore are less sensitive for agents such as clonazepam and lorazepam. The cutoff value is usually either 200 or 300 ng/mL, which can detect high doses but may not detect a therapeutic dose, resulting in a false-negative result.

Urine detection times generally range from 2 to 4 days, depending on the benzodiazepine. False-positive results are infrequent but can be seen with sertraline and efavirenz (Saitman et al. 2014). Other types of toxicology screening are also available (serum, hair, oral fluid, sweat) but are typically used in forensic or workplace settings.

TABLE 6–2. Equivalent doses and half-lives of commonly used benzodiazepines

Benzodiazepine	Time to peak concentration (hours)	Half-life (hours)	Typical frequency	Equivalency (mg)
Alprazolam	1–2	12–15	Three times a day	0.5–1
Lorazepam	1–2	10–20	Three or four times a day	2
Clonazepam	1–4	18–50	Three times a day	1–2
Oxazepam	3	5–11	Three or four times a day	10–15
Chlordiazepoxide	Several	24–48	Three or four times a day	25
Diazepam	0.5–6	20–80	Three or four times a day	10

How to Recognize Intoxication

CLINICAL PICTURE

Note that mild to moderate symptoms of intoxication, including impaired attention and anterograde amnesia, can be seen even at less than therapeutic doses. Severe intoxication, typically in the elderly, can result in paradoxical agitation. Additional features of benzodiazepine intoxication are included in the DSM-5 criteria for sedative, hypnotic, or anxiolytic intoxication (American Psychiatric Association 2013; Box 6–1).

Box 6–1.   Diagnostic Criteria for Sedative, Hypnotic, or Anxiolytic Intoxication

---

A. Recent use of a sedative, hypnotic, or anxiolytic.

B. Clinically significant maladaptive behavioral or psychological changes (e.g., inappropriate sexual or aggressive behavior, mood lability, impaired judgment) that developed during, or shortly after, sedative, hypnotic, or anxiolytic use.

C. One (or more) of the following signs or symptoms developing during, or shortly after, sedative, hypnotic, or anxiolytic use:

   1. Slurred speech.
   2. Incoordination.
   3. Unsteady gait.
   4. Nystagmus.
   5. Impairment in cognition (e.g., attention, memory).
   6. Stupor or coma.

D. The signs or symptoms are not attributable to another medical condition and are not better explained by another mental disorder, including intoxication with another substance.

OBTAINING THE HISTORY

The clinician must qualify benzodiazepine use (type of drug, amount, method of use, last use) and be aware of any concurrent alcohol or drug use. He or she should collect collateral information from family, friends, or medical records.

TOLERANCE

In general, tolerance is most rapid for shorter-acting, higher-potency agents such as alprazolam. Tolerance develops for the anticonvulsant effects, which limits long-term management of seizures with benzodiazepines. Rapid escalation of dosage can occur when benzodiazepines are used for insomnia because tolerance for sedation occurs quickly. Although tolerance does not develop for the anxiolytic properties, some patients may associate improvement of anxiety with the medication only and feel compelled to use the agent for relief instead of other coping skills. In addition, patients may misinterpret withdrawal anxiety as return of symptoms, resulting in the use of higher doses.

What to Do About Intoxication

CNS depression is the primary concern. If the patient appears sedated with decreased respiration, he or she should be monitored in a medical setting. Benzodiazepine use alone is a rare cause of overdose death; most patients improve with supportive treatment. Initially, the airway must be protected and ventilation provided as necessary. Also, it may be possible to use activated charcoal to evacuate the stomach contents.

Flumazenil is a competitive $GABA_A$ receptor antagonist used to reverse the effects of a benzodiazepine overdose. Initially, no more than 1 mg of intravenous flumazenil is given slowly. The half-life of flumazenil is 30–60 minutes, so it is important to observe for recurrence of intoxication. Patients who have used longer-acting benzodiazepines such as diazepam may need a flumazenil infusion and continuous monitoring. Flumazenil stimulates the upregulation of GABA receptors and reverses the uncoupling of benzodiazepines to the $GABA_A$ receptors. All patients should be observed closely after flumazenil is administered given the elevated risk of seizures and cardiac arrhythmias, which limits its liberal use.

MEDICAL WORKUP

The clinician should rule out hypoglycemia, fluid and electrolyte abnormalities, and any other potential etiologies for an altered mental status relevant to the patient's history and presentation. He or she must obtain a toxicology screen and a blood alcohol level and consider concurrent intoxication with another substance. Opioid use is common among benzodiazepine-using individuals and may not be detectable on a urine toxicology screen; naloxone can be used to reverse overdose. Naloxone is inactive in the absence of opioids and is therefore a safe intervention that should be used if opioid use is suspected.

How to Recognize Withdrawal

Clinically significant withdrawal is most likely to occur following daily use for at least 4–6 months (low dose) or 2–3 months (high dose). In intoxication, benzodiazepines suppress CNS function by potentiating GABAergic inhibition. In withdrawal, the absence of benzodiazepines leads to CNS hyperactivity secondary to decreased GABAergic inhibition along with increased glutamatergic response. DSM-5 criteria for sedative, hypnotic, or anxiolytic withdrawal (Box 6–2) are to be used in the diagnosis of benzodiazepine withdrawal.

Rebound withdrawal is usually more intense, of shorter duration, and self-limited. Pseudowithdrawal is overinterpretation of symptoms secondary to the expectation of withdrawal.

Box 6–2.   Diagnostic Criteria for Sedative, Hypnotic, or Anxiolytic Withdrawal

---

A. Cessation of (or reduction in) sedative, hypnotic, or anxiolytic use that has been prolonged.

B. Two (or more) of the following, developing within several hours to a few days after the cessation of (or reduction in) sedative, hypnotic, or anxiolytic use described in Criterion A:

1. Autonomic hyperactivity (e.g., sweating or pulse rate greater than 100 bpm).
2. Hand tremor.
3. Insomnia.
4. Nausea or vomiting.
5. Transient visual, tactile, or auditory hallucinations or illusions.
6. Psychomotor agitation.
7. Anxiety.
8. Grand mal seizures.

C. The signs or symptoms in Criterion B cause clinically significant distress or impairment in social, occupational, or other important areas of functioning.

D. The signs or symptoms are not attributable to another medical condition and are not better explained by another mental disorder, including intoxication or withdrawal from another substance.

Specify if:
   With perceptual disturbances

Benzodiazepines

Benzodiazepine withdrawal has two phases:

1. **Acute withdrawal** (hours to days) tends to be seen in patients who have used higher than therapeutic doses for more than 1 month and is associated with typical and dangerous symptoms, including tremors, seizures, and delirium. Acute withdrawal must be recognized early to prevent complications.
2. **Protracted abstinence syndrome** (weeks to months) tends to be seen in patients who have taken therapeutic doses for at least 3 months. These symptoms are often confused with return of the original symptomatology because they manifest as anxiety, insomnia, and cognitive impairment. The psychological discomfort and increased benzodiazepine cravings are thought to contribute significantly to high relapse rates. If symptoms do not resolve, the clinician should consider a psychological component or comorbid psychiatric disorder.

The severity of withdrawal depends on the type and dose of benzodiazepine, along with the duration of use. In general, withdrawal is worse for shorter-acting, higher-potency agents such as alprazolam. Onset for short-acting agents (i.e., alprazolam, lorazepam, oxazepam) can occur within 24 hours, peaking at 1–5 days, and lasting for 7–21 days. Onset for longer-acting agents (i.e., clonazepam, chlordiazepoxide, diazepam) can occur within 5 days, peaking at 1–9 days, and lasting 10–28 days.

The risk of withdrawal is greater in patients who have been taking higher doses of benzodiazepines over a longer period of time. Those with psychiatric or medical comorbidity, as well as those currently using or withdrawing from other substances, tend to have a more complicated withdrawal. Allowing patients to go through untreated benzodiazepine withdrawal is not recommended during acute medical or surgical hospitalizations.

Benzodiazepine use peaks at ages 65–80. Given that cytochrome P450 metabolism decreases with age, older individuals are more likely to experience a protracted withdrawal. Women are prescribed benzodiazepines twice as often as men and typically have more intense withdrawal (Olfson et al. 2015).

What to Do About Withdrawal

Dosage and withdrawal scales should be individualized for each patient. Geriatric patients should start with lower doses of benzodiazepines than those used for younger adults. The Clinical Institute Withdrawal Assessment—Benzodiazepines can be used to assess for acute withdrawal symptoms. The first symptom is often anxiety.

The following are two typical treatment strategies for withdrawal:

1. **Substitution then tapering:** for patients taking a shorter-acting benzodiazepine, substitute a longer-acting benzodiazepine at an equivalent dose such as chlordiazepoxide or clonazepam. Oxazepam can be used in patients with hepatic impairment; it is preferred to lorazepam given lorazepam's higher abuse potential.
2. **Simple tapering:** gradually decrease the dosage of the agent the patient is currently taking.

The rate of systematic discontinuation is contingent on the individual, dose, and duration of use. Inpatient treatment should be considered for patients with polysubstance dependence, high-dose use, psychiatric comorbidity, or erratic behavior. Inpatients are most likely in a detoxification setting with a set protocol that will typically reduce the dose by 10% each day. For outpatients, the taper is more gradual, with decreases typically occurring at 10% per week or two. Regardless of setting, the taper schedule should be evaluated throughout to ensure that the rate is clinically appropriate and safe. Typically, the first half of the taper is the easiest and quickest, allowing for bigger and more rapid cuts.

In addition to benzodiazepines, adjunct medication is occasionally used, such as carbamazepine, divalproex sodium, propranolol, or trazodone.

How to Recognize Addiction

A nonjudgmental disposition is critical to accurately assess any substance use disorder. Rapport can be quickly built by sitting at eye level, maintaining eye contact, engaging fully, and relaying empathy throughout the encounter.

Approximately 1 in 20 U.S. adults filled at least one prescription for a benzodiazepine in 2008; this does not include illegally obtained benzodiazepines. The highest rate of use was among 80-year-old women (Olfson et al. 2015).

The rate of development of physiological dependence is contingent on the pharmacological properties of the agent, the dose, the duration of use, and the individual. Diazepam and alprazolam have a higher abuse potential given greater lipid solubility and faster onset of action, as compared with chlordiazepoxide or oxazepam. Tolerance and withdrawal phenomena are common with chronic benzodiazepine use. As shown in the DSM-5 criteria for sedative, hypnotic, or anxiolytic use disorder (Box 6–3), benzodiazepine use disorder should be diagnosed when additional signs are present. DSM-5 specifies levels of severity depending on the number of criteria met.

Box 6–3.   Diagnostic Criteria for Sedative, Hypnotic, or Anxiolytic Use Disorder

---

A. A problematic pattern of sedative, hypnotic, or anxiolytic use leading to clinically significant impairment or distress, as manifested by at least two of the following, occurring within a 12-month period:

1. Sedatives, hypnotics, or anxiolytics are often taken in larger amounts or over a longer period than was intended.
2. There is a persistent desire or unsuccessful efforts to cut down or control sedative, hypnotic, or anxiolytic use.
3. A great deal of time is spent in activities necessary to obtain the sedative, hypnotic, or anxiolytic; use the sedative, hypnotic, or anxiolytic; or recover from its effects.
4. Craving, or a strong desire or urge to use the sedative, hypnotic, or anxiolytic.
5. Recurrent sedative, hypnotic, or anxiolytic use resulting in a failure to fulfill major role obligations at work, school, or home (e.g., repeated absences from work or poor work performance related to sedative, hypnotic, or anxiolytic use; sedative-, hypnotic-, or anxiolytic-related absences, suspensions, or expulsions from school; neglect of children or household).
6. Continued sedative, hypnotic, or anxiolytic use despite having persistent or recurrent social or interpersonal problems caused or exacerbated by the effects of sedatives, hypnotics, or anxiolytics (e.g., arguments with a spouse about consequences of intoxication; physical fights).
7. Important social, occupational, or recreational activities are given up or reduced because of sedative, hypnotic, or anxiolytic use.

8. Recurrent sedative, hypnotic, or anxiolytic use in situations in which it is physically hazardous (e.g., driving an automobile or operating a machine when impaired by sedative, hypnotic, or anxiolytic use).

9. Sedative, hypnotic, or anxiolytic use is continued despite knowledge of having a persistent or recurrent physical or psychological problem that is likely to have been caused or exacerbated by the sedative, hypnotic, or anxiolytic.

10. Tolerance, as defined by either of the following:

    a. A need for markedly increased amounts of the sedative, hypnotic, or anxiolytic to achieve intoxication or desired effect.

    b. A markedly diminished effect with continued use of the same amount of the sedative, hypnotic, or anxiolytic.

    Note: This criterion is not considered to be met for individuals taking sedatives, hypnotics, or anxiolytics under medical supervision.

11. Withdrawal, as manifested by either of the following:

    a. The characteristic withdrawal syndrome for sedatives, hypnotics, or anxiolytics (refer to Criteria A and B of the criteria set for sedative, hypnotic, or anxiolytic withdrawal).

    b. Sedatives, hypnotics, or anxiolytics (or a closely related substance, such as alcohol) are taken to relieve or avoid withdrawal symptoms.

    Note: This criterion is not considered to be met for individuals taking sedatives, hypnotics, or anxiolytics under medical supervision.

Specify if:
In early remission
In sustained remission

Specify if:
In a controlled environment

Specify current severity:
Mild: Presence of 2–3 symptoms.
Moderate: Presence of 4–5 symptoms.
Severe: Presence of 6 or more symptoms.

Clinicians who suspect a benzodiazepine use disorder should consider additional screening areas: other substance use, depression, anxiety, the safety of the patient with regard to living situation, and personal relationships.

What to Do About Addiction

Currently, neither maintenance treatment nor chronic antagonist therapy are options for benzodiazepine use disorders. Supervised detoxification is recommended. Alternative agents may be used to address the underlying anxiety (SSRIs, buspirone, anticonvulsants, antihypertensives, tricyclic antidepressants, atypical antipsychotics, hydroxyzine) and insomnia (trazodone, mirtazapine, tricyclic antidepressants, melatonin agonists, antihistamines). Zolpidem should be avoided given its abuse potential.

Pharmacotherapy alone is rarely sufficient to treat a benzodiazepine use disorder. Patients also should be offered individual or group therapy, along with a referral to self-help groups such as Alcoholics Anonymous (AA) or Narcotics Anonymous (NA). Patients often need to try a few different groups to find the right fit and should be encouraged to do so. A patient who is unable to maintain sobriety likely requires a higher level of care, such as an intensive outpatient program or inpatient rehabilitation.

Serious overdose and death can occur if alcohol, benzodiazepines, sedatives, tranquilizers, or antidepressants are taken with methadone or buprenorphine. For patients with dependence on CNS depressants who are receiving opioid maintenance, clinicians should consider an opioid treatment program as opposed to office-based opioid treatment.

Special Issues With Psychiatric Comorbidities

Comorbid psychiatric disorders are common among patients with benzodiazepine use disorders. It is estimated that 2.6% of the patients with an anxiety disorder also have a sedative use disorder (Conway et al. 2006). Patients with an alcohol use disorder and/or opioid use disorder (especially those receiving maintenance therapy) are at much higher risk of misusing benzodiazepines and should be screened regularly.

An accurate diagnosis can be difficult because symptoms of withdrawal and intoxication often mimic psychiatric disorders, including personality disorders. Ideally, making a diagnosis should be postponed until a thorough history with collateral information is obtained and the clinician has had the opportunity to evaluate the patient during a period of abstinence. Untreated symptoms of anxiety or depression can lead to difficulty in engaging patients in treatment and therefore should be addressed. Note that benzodiazepines themselves can worsen depression, causing suicidal ideation in some patients.

In general, benzodiazepines should be avoided in patients with comorbid personality disorder (more specifically, borderline personality disorder or traits) because these agents can lead to further mood lability and disinhibition.

Special Issues With Medical Comorbidities

Benzodiazepine use can be associated with many medical complications. Benzodiazepines can produce significant respiratory depression when used in excess or combined with other CNS depressants. They should be used with caution in patients with pulmonary disease, including sleep apnea, because benzodiazepines can decrease muscle tone, leading to hypercarbia and associated complications. Although benzodiazepines increase total sleep time and decrease nighttime awakenings, they cause less time in stage 3 sleep, which is associated with restorative sleep (Mendelson 1987).

Special Issues With Specific Populations

PREGNANCY

Benzodiazepine use during pregnancy is a challenging problem, especially because patients may not feel comfortable disclosing their use for fear of stigma and legal or custody concerns; therefore, all patients should be screened appropriately. Benzodiazepines are Category D drugs. Historically there have been concerns about cleft lip or palate and urogenital and neurological malformations with use in the first trimester, although recent literature no longer supports this concern (Bellantuono et al. 2013).

Use should be minimized after weighing the risks and benefits. Clinicians should consider prescribing a shorter-acting agent, such as lorazepam, on an as-needed basis or initiating and maintaining patients on an antidepressant, typically Category C. Use near delivery should be limited to minimize withdrawal symptoms and associated low Apgar scores in the infant.

All benzodiazepines cross into breast milk, and long-term effects are unknown. Infants may develop floppy baby syndrome, which includes respiratory depression, sedation, and hypotonia. Because infants have not developed the mechanisms for metabolism, the half-life of benzodiazepines is typically longer than expected; therefore, a shorter-acting agent is preferred if a benzodiazepine is needed for patients who are breast-feeding.

PAIN

Management of pain in a benzodiazepine-dependent patient can be complex given the concurrent use of a CNS depressant. Although benzodiazepines are not typically used for direct pain relief, they are commonly used for associated muscle spasm, anxiety, and insomnia. These patients ideally would be managed by pain management specialists. Treatment of comorbid psychiatric issues is essential.

ELDERLY

Secondary to widely known changes in metabolism in the elderly, this patient population is particularly vulnerable to the effects of intoxication with and withdrawal from benzodiazepines. "In general, all benzodiazepines increase risk of cognitive impairment, delirium, falls, fractures, and motor vehicle accidents in older adults" (American Geriatrics Society 2015 Beers Criteria Update Expert Panel 2015, p. 7). Undiagnosed and untreated benzodiazepine use disorders can lead to significant morbidity and mortality. Discontinuation typically leads to improved cognition and motor ability and less anxiety.

KEY POINTS

Benzodiazepines are effective at relieving symptoms of anxiety and insomnia in the short term; however, the risks need to be carefully weighed against potential benefits. Although medically safe at therapeutic doses, benzodiazepine overdose when combined with other agents is associated with a high risk of death. Similar to patients taking opioids, patients taking benzodiazepines may have a false perception of minimal harm because these are prescription medications.

Benzodiazepines are considered first-line treatment for alcohol withdrawal. In general, if intravenous use is indicated, diazepam or lorazepam is recommended. If the patient is able to take medications by mouth and is in mild to moderate withdrawal, chlordiazepoxide should be considered; lorazepam or oxazepam should be used if the patient has liver impairment.

Prevention is the key; benzodiazepines should not be considered first-line treatment for anxiety or insomnia. In addition to behavioral interventions, SSRIs and non-addictive agents are recommended. Avoid sedative-hypnotic use in the elderly. If benzodiazepines are used as an adjunct, it should be for weeks, not months or years.

If the patient is able to take medications orally, a longer-acting agent such as clonazepam rather than lorazepam should be considered. Medication regimens should be reviewed periodically to ensure ongoing medical necessity, especially for the most vulnerable population: elderly women. If long-term use is deemed appropriate, the dose should be tapered to maximize effect but minimize side effects.

References

American Geriatrics Society 2015 Beers Criteria Update Expert Panel: American Geriatrics Society 2015 Updated Beers Criteria for Potentially Inappropriate Medication Use in Older Adults. J Am Geriatr Soc 63(11):2227–2246, 2015 26446832

American Psychiatric Association: Diagnostic and Statistical Manual of Mental Disorders, 5th Edition. Arlington, VA, American Psychiatric Association, 2013

Bellantuono C, Tofani S, Di Sciascio G, et al: Benzodiazepine exposure in pregnancy and risk of major malformations: a critical overview. Gen Hosp Psychiatry 35(1):3–8, 2013 23044244

Billioti de Gage S, Moride Y, Ducruet T, et al: Benzodiazepine use and risk of Alzheimer's disease: case-control study. BMJ 349:g5205, 2014 25208536

Conway KP, Compton W, Stinson FS, et al: Lifetime comorbidity of DSM-IV mood and anxiety disorders and specific drug use disorders: results from the National Epidemiologic Survey on Alcohol and Related Conditions. J Clin Psychiatry 67(2):247–257, 2006 16566620

Mendelson WB: Human Sleep: Research and Clinical Care. New York, Plenum, 1987

Olfson M, King M, Schoenbaum M: Benzodiazepine use in the United States. JAMA Psychiatry 72(2):136–142, 2015

Olsen RW, Betz H: GABA and glycine, in Basic Neurochemistry: Molecular, Cellular and Medical Aspects, 7th Edition. Edited by Siegel GJ, Albers RW, Brady S, et al. New York, Elsevier, 2006, pp 291–302

Saitman A, Park HD, Fitzgerald RL: False-positive interferences of common urine drug screen immunoassays: a review. J Anal Toxicol 38(7):387–396, 2014 24986836

CHAPTER 7

Caffeine

GRACE HENNESSY, M.D.

FOUND in the fruit, beans, and leaves of more than 60 plants, caffeine has been used in various forms by different cultures for centuries. The most common natural sources of caffeine are coffee beans, tea, cocoa, guarana, kola nuts, and yerba maté. Today, caffeine is added to a variety of foods, ranging from yogurt to energy drinks to over-the-counter and prescription medications. Table 7–1 lists the caffeine content of a representative sample of food items and medications. With so many different forms of caffeine available, it is no surprise that caffeine is the most widely consumed legal substance today.

Pharmacology

Caffeine (1,3,7-trimethylxanthine) is an odorless, bitter, white crystalline alkaloid of the methylxanthine family. Orally ingested caffeine is rapidly absorbed into the bloodstream and passes quickly through the blood-brain barrier. Caffeine blood concentrations peak about 30–45 minutes after ingestion, and the half-life is approximately 4–6 hours. Caffeine is primarily metabolized in the liver by cytochrome P450 (CYP) 1A2 into the active metabolites paraxanthine, theophylline, and theobromide. In the central nervous system, caffeine acts as a nonselective antagonist at the adenosine receptors A_1 and A_2. Adenosine, a purine nucleoside, suppresses neuronal activity, and this effect is blocked when caffeine reversibly binds to adenosine receptors. Caffeine also increases dopaminergic neuronal activity by removing the inhibitory effect adenosine exerts at dopamine receptors. This change in dopamine activity is associated with the rewarding aspects of caffeine. By blocking adenosine receptors, caffeine causes

TABLE 7–1. Caffeine content of a representative sample of beverages, foods, and medications

Source and serving size	Typical caffeine content (mg)
Coffee	
Decaffeinated, 12 oz	8
Espresso, 1 oz	70
Instant, 12 oz	140
Brewed or drip, 12 oz	200
Tea	
Herbal, brewed, 8 oz	0
Instant, 6 oz	30
Brewed, 6 oz	40
Soft drinks	
Sprite, 7-Up, and ginger ale, 12 oz	0
Coca-Cola, 12 oz	35
Pepsi, 12 oz	38
Mountain Dew, 12 oz	55
Energy drinks	
Red Bull, 8.3 oz	80
Monster Energy and Rockstar, 16 oz	160
5-Hour Energy, 2 oz	215
Food	
Hershey's Milk Chocolate bar, 1.55 oz	9
Hershey's Special Dark, 1.45 oz	20
Dannon coffee low-fat yogurt, 6 oz	30
Over-the-counter stimulants	
No-Doz or Vivarin, 1 caplet	200
Over-the-counter weight loss products	
Hydroxycut and Dexatrim, 2 caplets	200

TABLE 7–1. Caffeine content of a representative sample of beverages, foods, and medications *(continued)*

Source and serving size	Typical caffeine content (mg)
Pain relievers	
Anacin, 2 tablets	64
Fiorinal and Fioricet, 2 tablets	80
Excedrin Extra Strength, 2 tablets	130
Cafergot, 2 tablets	200
Caffeine anhydrous	
Powder, 1/16 teaspoon	200
Powder, 1 teaspoon	3,200

Source. Adapted from Juliano et al. 2014.

- Increased neuronal firing
- Increased turnover of neurotransmitters such as norepinephrine and acetylcholine
- Inhibition of sleep
- Cerebral vasoconstriction

In the periphery, caffeine use results in

- Increased blood pressure
- Increased heart rate
- Relaxation of bronchial smooth muscle
- Increased gastric secretion
- Increased urinary output

Caffeine consumption in doses of 200 mg (approximately two cups of coffee) or less is associated with the following positive subjective effects:

- Increased wakefulness
- Improved attention
- Improved reaction time
- Increased sense of well-being
- Increased sociability

At doses higher than 200 mg, however, caffeine has been shown to cause several negative subjective effects:

- Anxiety, nervousness, and jitteriness
- Irritability
- Gastrointestinal discomfort
- Insomnia

Note that the negative subjective effects of caffeine could occur at doses lower than 200 mg in children, older adults, caffeine-naive individuals, and those who are sensitive to its effects.

TOXICOLOGY

Standard and extended urine drug tests do not test for caffeine. Caffeine metabolites are excreted in the urine and can be quantified through high-performance liquid chromatography–mass spectrometry.

How to Recognize Intoxication

Box 7–1 contains DSM-5 criteria for caffeine intoxication (American Psychiatric Association 2013). Caffeine intoxication generally occurs after ingestion of amounts greater than 250 mg, as described in DSM-5 Criteria B1–B7. At doses of 1 g/day or higher, other caffeine intoxication symptoms may emerge, as described in DSM-5 Criteria B8–B12.

Box 7–1. Diagnostic Criteria for Caffeine Intoxication

A. Recent consumption of caffeine (typically a high dose well in excess of 250 mg).
B. Five (or more) of the following signs or symptoms developing during, or shortly after, caffeine use:
    1. Restlessness.
    2. Nervousness.
    3. Excitement.
    4. Insomnia.
    5. Flushed face.
    6. Diuresis.
    7. Gastrointestinal disturbance.

8. Muscle twitching.
9. Rambling flow of thought and speech.
10. Tachycardia or cardiac arrhythmia.
11. Periods of inexhaustibility.
12. Psychomotor agitation.

C. The signs or symptoms in Criterion B cause clinically significant distress or impairment in social, occupational, or other important areas of functioning.

D. The signs or symptoms are not attributable to another medical condition and are not better explained by another mental disorder, including intoxication with another substance.

The lethal dose of caffeine for adults is estimated to be 10 g. Death from caffeine overdose is usually proceeded by

- Abdominal pain
- Vomiting
- Extreme tachycardia
- Severe agitation
- Seizures

OBTAINING THE HISTORY

The history should include the amount of caffeine consumed as well as the form in which it was ingested (i.e., coffee, energy drink, powder). Other relevant information, including current and past medical problems, psychiatric conditions, current medications, and other substance use, also should be obtained. Psychiatric syndromes and disorders that are similar to caffeine intoxication include mania; panic attack; akathisia; sleep disorders; generalized anxiety disorder; stimulant intoxication; sedative, hypnotic, or anxiolytic withdrawal; and tobacco withdrawal.

What to Do About Intoxication

Symptoms of intoxication associated with low doses of caffeine usually resolve spontaneously within 1 day and do not require medical intervention. Caffeine overdose, however, should be treated in an emergency medical setting and may involve intubation and mechanical ventilation to protect the airway, charcoal administration or gastric lavage to expedite caffeine removal from the gastrointestinal tract, intravenous fluids to support circulation, and medications to manage cardiac arrhythmias and seizures.

MEDICAL WORKUP

Thyrotoxicosis can resemble caffeine toxicity and should be ruled out with thyroid function tests. Routine blood tests in caffeine overdose will identify hypokalemia, hyperglycemia, and an increased anion gap. Because caffeine is found in prescription and over-the-counter analgesics, toxicology testing should include acetaminophen, salicylates, and barbiturates to determine whether treatment for toxic levels of these substances is also necessary.

How to Recognize Withdrawal

Similar to other substances of abuse, habitual caffeine use can result in tolerance and withdrawal. Indeed, tolerance to some of the subjective and physiological effects of caffeine has been observed in animals and humans after daily consumption. Box 7–2 contains DSM-5 criteria for caffeine withdrawal.

Box 7–2. Diagnostic Criteria for Caffeine Withdrawal

A. Prolonged daily use of caffeine.

B. Abrupt cessation of or reduction in caffeine use, followed within 24 hours by three (or more) of the following signs or symptoms:

1. Headache.
2. Marked fatigue or drowsiness.
3. Dysphoric mood, depressed mood, or irritability.
4. Difficulty concentrating.
5. Flu-like symptoms (nausea, vomiting, or muscle pain/ stiffness).

C. The signs or symptoms in Criterion B cause clinically significant distress or impairment in social, occupational, or other important areas of functioning.

D. The signs or symptoms are not associated with the physiological effects of another medical condition (e.g., migraine, viral illness) and are not better explained by another mental disorder, including intoxication or withdrawal from another substance.

The severity of caffeine withdrawal is usually related to the daily amount of caffeine consumed. Symptoms begin about 12–24 hours after the last dose of caffeine, peak at about 20–50 hours, and can last from 2 to 9 days. Headaches are considered the hallmark sign of caffeine withdrawal and can last up to 21 days. Headaches are likely a result of rebound cerebral vasodilation and increased cerebral blood flow.

What to Do About Withdrawal

Although uncomfortable, caffeine withdrawal is not life-threatening and will resolve in time without any specific interventions. For intolerable withdrawal symptoms, introducing lower doses of caffeine than those typically consumed can lessen symptom severity. Symptoms of caffeine withdrawal usually resolve within 30–60 minutes after caffeine is consumed again. The best way to decrease the likelihood of caffeine withdrawal is to decrease gradually the daily amount of caffeine ingested over days or weeks rather than to stop consuming caffeine abruptly.

How to Recognize Addiction

Caffeine use disorder is not included in the main body of "Substance-Related and Addictive Disorders" in DSM-5, but it is included in Section III, in "Conditions for Further Study," as shown in Box 7–3. Severity levels (i.e., mild, moderate, and severe) based on the number of proposed criteria present have not been established.

Box 7–3.   Proposed Criteria for Caffeine Use Disorder

A problematic pattern of caffeine use leading to clinically significant impairment or distress, as manifested by at least the first three of the following criteria occurring within a 12-month period:

1. A persistent desire or unsuccessful efforts to cut down or control caffeine use.
2. Continued caffeine use despite knowledge of having a persistent or recurrent physical or psychological problem that is likely to have been caused or exacerbated by caffeine.
3. Withdrawal, as manifested by either of the following:
   a. The characteristic withdrawal syndrome for caffeine.
   b. Caffeine (or a closely related) substance is taken to relieve or avoid withdrawal symptoms.

4. Caffeine is often taken in larger amounts or over a longer period than was intended.
5. Recurrent caffeine use resulting in a failure to fulfill major role obligations at work, school, or home (e.g., repeated tardiness or absences from work or school related to caffeine use or withdrawal).
6. Continued caffeine use despite having persistent or recurrent social or interpersonal problems caused or exacerbated by the effects of caffeine (e.g., arguments with spouse about consequences of use, medical problems, cost).
7. Tolerance, as defined by either of the following:
   a. A need for markedly increased amounts of caffeine to achieve desired effect.
   b. Markedly diminished effect with continued use of the same amount of caffeine.
8. A great deal of time is spent in activities necessary to obtain caffeine, use caffeine, or recover from its effects.
9. Craving or a strong desire or urge to use caffeine.

The current prevalence of caffeine use disorder is not well defined. When the three required criteria and the tolerance criteria for caffeine use disorder are used, the prevalence is approximately 9% of current caffeine consumers. This number rises to 20% in pain clinic patients who have a recent history of substance misuse, in high school and college students, and among individuals in drug treatment who are considered to be at a higher risk for developing the disorder.

What to Do About Addiction

No validated empirical pharmacological or psychosocial treatments for caffeine use disorder are currently available. Strategies for reducing or ending caffeine use have been adapted from other behavioral treatments for tobacco and other substance-related disorders. These strategies include

- Education about the sources of caffeine
- Caffeine self-monitoring through a food diary
- Calculating daily caffeine intake
- Establishing a caffeine modification goal
- Creating a gradual reduction schedule
- Using behavioral modification strategies such as social support
- Follow-up with a clinician such as a primary care provider to monitor progress

Although there is no single, well-defined reduction schedule for all individuals with excessive caffeine use, gradual reductions that occur over the course of 3–4 weeks have been shown to be effective. Data on relapse rates to caffeine use are not available.

Special Issues With Psychiatric Comorbidities

Caffeine has been shown to worsen anxiety symptoms in those diagnosed with panic disorder, generalized anxiety disorder, or performance social anxiety disorder. Caffeine, when consumed in high doses, also may precipitate mania and induce or exacerbate psychotic symptoms in individuals with paranoid traits or schizophrenia. Low or moderate coffee consumption in the range of two to six cups per day may lower the risk of suicide, but consumption of greater than eight cups per day has been associated with an increased risk. Lastly, symptoms of caffeine use disorder such as tolerance and withdrawal have been positively associated with major depression; antisocial personality disorder; and alcohol, cannabis, and cocaine use disorders.

Special Issues With Medical Comorbidities

Caffeinated and decaffeinated coffee contain lipids that increase total cholesterol and low-density lipoprotein. Elevations in blood pressure that persist for several hours after caffeine consumption also have been documented. Caffeine is associated with variations in heart rate and arterial stiffness soon after consumption. The implications of these coffee- or caffeine-induced effects on long-term health are not entirely clear and need more study.

Cancers of the bladder, pancreas, and ovaries were reportedly associated with caffeine consumption, but controlled studies have failed to show an association. No clear evidence shows that caffeine-related increases in urinary calcium excretion are associated with osteoporosis or bone fractures in women. Evidence does suggest that caffeine may be associated with a reduced risk of Parkinson's disease, Alzheimer's disease, and gallstones. Coffee drinking may reduce the incidence of chronic liver disease and type 2 diabetes, but these effects may be a result of compounds in coffee other than caffeine.

Special Issues With Specific Populations

PREGNANCY

Caffeine freely passes through the placenta and is disseminated throughout fetal tissues. Maternal caffeine metabolism decreases and fetal caffeine exposure increases as a pregnancy progresses. Additionally, the developing fetus lacks the enzymes necessary to break down caffeine, and caffeine metabolites have been found to collect in the fetal brain. The American College of Obstetricians and Gynecologists (2010) recommend that pregnant women consume no more than 200 mg/day of caffeine, the equivalent of one 12-ounce cup of brewed coffee.

Caffeine use during pregnancy has been associated with negative outcomes, such as an increased rate of spontaneous abortion, preterm labor, intrauterine growth retardation, decreased birth weight, and small for gestational age. The evidence for these conditions is conflicting, and more study is needed to determine what effects caffeine has on pregnancy outcomes.

CHILDREN, ADOLESCENTS, AND YOUNG ADULTS

Approximately 73% of children, adolescents, and young adults consume caffeine in some form each day (Branum et al. 2014). Although soda remains their primary source of caffeine, the percentage of youths consuming soda has decreased over time, whereas the percentage consuming coffee and energy drinks has steadily increased. The increase in energy drink consumption in recent years mirrors an increase in emergency department visits by 18- to 25-year-olds who report caffeine-related adverse events such as nausea, vomiting, tachycardia, agitation, and chest pain after consuming energy drinks (Reissig et al. 2009).

Another concern is the consumption of alcohol mixed with energy drinks. By offsetting the sedating effects of alcohol, the high levels of caffeine in energy drinks may reduce consumers' subjective feelings of intoxication, which can impair their judgment about risky behaviors because they do not believe that they are drunk. Negative consequences associated with alcohol mixed with energy drinks include approximately double the risk of requiring medical treatment, committing or being the victim of sexual assault, riding with an intoxicated driver, and having an alcohol-related motor vehicle accident (Howland and Rohsenow 2013).

The use of pure powdered caffeine, also known as *caffeine anhydrous,* has become popular among teenagers and young adults as a way to boost athletic performance, lose weight, and increase energy. Caffeine powder is sold in bulk bags on the Internet without clear instructions about its use. A full tablespoon of caffeine powder contains 3,200 mg of caffeine, the equivalent of sixteen 12-ounce cups of brewed or drip coffee. Serious adverse medical events and deaths from the overuse of caffeine powder by adolescents and young adults have been reported.

KEY POINTS

Caffeine has been consumed around the world for centuries. In doses of 200 mg or less, caffeine is associated with increased alertness, improved reaction time, increased sense of well-being, and sociability. Higher doses have been associated with anxiety, irritability, gastrointestinal distress, and tachycardia. Toxic doses of caffeine have been associated with serious medical outcomes such as cardiac arrhythmias, seizure, and death.

Regular caffeine consumption results in the development of dependence, with tolerance and withdrawal cited as common symptoms.

No empirically validated treatments for caffeine dependence are available, but the reintroduction of caffeine will reverse withdrawal symptoms, and gradual decreases in caffeine use over time rather than abrupt cessation may ameliorate symptoms of caffeine withdrawal.

Behavioral interventions such as those used for the treatment of substance-related disorders might help individuals achieve abstinence from caffeine.

The effects of caffeine on various medical conditions are not well defined and require more study. Caffeine use increases anxiety in individuals with underlying anxiety disorders and may induce mania or psychosis in susceptible individuals. Caffeine use may lower suicide risk and the risk of developing Parkinson's disease and Alzheimer's disease.

Energy drink use among adolescents and young adults is a growing concern and has been associated with an increase in adverse medical events and emergency department visits in this cohort. Alcohol mixed with energy drinks may lead to increased risk-taking activities among youth, and the use of pure powder caffeine can result in serious medical consequences and even death.

References

American College of Obstetricians and Gynecologists: ACOG Committee Opinion No. 462: Moderate caffeine consumption during pregnancy. Obstet Gynecol 116(2 Pt 1):467–468, 2010 20664420

American Psychiatric Association: Diagnostic and Statistical Manual of Mental Disorders, 5th Edition. Arlington, VA, American Psychiatric Association, 2013

Branum AM, Rossen LM, Schoendorf KC: Trends in caffeine intake among U.S. children and adolescents. Pediatrics 133(3):386–393, 2014 24515508

Howland J, Rohsenow DJ: Risks of energy drinks mixed with alcohol. JAMA 309(3):245–246, 2013 23330172

Juliano LM, Ferré S, Griffiths RR: The pharmacology of caffeine, in The ASAM Principles of Addiction Medicine, 5th Edition. Edited by Ries RK, Fiellin DA, Miller SC, et al. Philadelphia, PA, Lippincott Williams & Wilkins, 2014, pp 180–200

Reissig CJ, Strain EC, Griffiths RR: Caffeinated energy drinks—a growing problem. Drug Alcohol Depend 99(1–3):1–10, 2009 18809264

CHAPTER 8

Cannabis

MICHAEL A. KETTERINGHAM, M.D., M.P.H.

CANNABIS is the most commonly used illegal substance in the United States, and the proportion of U.S. citizens who use cannabis has remained stable for the past 20 years despite increases in its potency and federal penalties aimed to restrict its use (Substance Abuse and Mental Health Services Administration Center for Behavioral Health Statistics and Quality 2014). Recently, the use of synthetic cannabinoids arose as a legal alternative to cannabis. In contrast to prohibitive federal law that relies mainly on penalizing cannabis users, at the time of this writing, more than 20 states have decriminalized medicinal marijuana and four states have legalized the possession and distribution of cannabis. The changing legal environment may increase the availability of cannabis, but it may also increase the availability of treatment while reducing the social consequences of high rates of imprisonment.

Pharmacology

The cannabis plant consists of more than 400 chemical compounds, of which approximately 60 cannabinoids have been identified. Tetrahydrocannabinol (THC) is the primary compound thought to produce the psychoactive effects referred to as the *high* and can be anxiogenic. Another well-studied compound, cannabidiol, is believed to produce an anxiolytic effect.

Cannabis is cultivated in nearly every country in the world and is processed into drug products with varying THC content. The whole plant contains approximately 1%–5% THC, unfertilized flowers 7%–15%, hashish or resin 10%–20%, and hash oil 20%–60%. In the United States, THC content in drug products has increased significantly since the 1960s.

Methods of cannabis administration vary the bioavailability of THC. Smoking or vaporizing cannabis has a bioavailability of approximately 10%–35%; intoxication occurs at 1 minute, with peak intensity at 15–30 minutes, persisting for approximately 4 hours. Oral intake has a bioavailability of 5%–20%; intoxication occurs at 30 minutes, with peak intensity at 2–3 hours, persisting up to 12 hours.

Once administered, THC is highly protein bound. Because of its lipophilic nature, THC crosses the blood-brain barrier to bind to central cannabinoid receptors. There are five endogenous ligands and two known receptor subtypes: CB_1 and CB_2. CB_1 is abundant but expressed in highest concentrations in the basal ganglia (reward, learning, motor control), cerebellum (sensorimotor coordination), hippocampus (memory), and cortex (planning, inhibition, higher-order cognition). CB_2 is found peripherally in immune system tissue and may modify immune response and inflammatory reactions. Table 8–1 links proposed CB_1 receptor locations with resulting symptoms of cannabis intoxication. Imaging has shown that changes in brain areas that express CB_1 occur in a THC dose- and time-dependent fashion.

THC also has been shown to increase dopamine neuronal firing and synaptic levels of dopamine, suggesting THC's involvement in the mesolimbic reward pathway (Ross and Peselow 2009). Animal studies have reported conditioned placed preference and self-administration that is prevented or reversed in CB_1 knockouts or those treated with CB_1 antagonists. Taken together, there is neurobiological and behavioral evidence of the addictive properties of cannabis. Furthermore, multiple studies have established that genetic influences contribute to the development of cannabis use disorders.

THC is metabolized in the liver to 11-OH-THC and THC-COOH (THC carboxylic acid) and then excreted into the urine and feces. Because of its lipophilicity, THC is distributed widely in the body and has an extended half-life of 25–36 hours. Presence of cannabinoid metabolites can be tested in urine, blood, oral fluid, sweat, and hair samples. Urine drug screen results remain positive for months past abstinence in the chronic heavy user, 2–4 weeks in the heavy user, and 7–10 days in the casual user. Thus, urine drug testing can establish only past use and cannot be used to diagnose acute intoxication.

TABLE 8–1. Cannabinoid receptor subtype CB_1 location and expected clinical manifestations of tetrahydrocannabinol activity

CB_1 receptor location	Clinical manifestations
Cerebral cortex	Altered consciousness, perceptual distortions, memory impairment, delusions, hallucinations
Hypothalamus	Increased appetite
Brain stem	Antiemetic, tachycardia, reduced blood pressure, drowsiness, pain reduction, reduced spasticity, reduced tremor
Basal ganglia	Slowed reaction time
Cerebellum	Reduced spasticity, impaired coordination
Hippocampus	Memory impairment
Nucleus accumbens	Motivation and reward
Amygdala	Increased or decreased anxiety, increased or decreased panic
Spinal cord	Altered pain sensitivity

How to Recognize Intoxication

Cannabis intoxication has both characteristic psychological and physiological symptoms. Psychological symptoms can vary. Intoxication can be enjoyable and relaxing for the user, increasing sociability and exaggerating visual and auditory perceptions while distorting the sense of time. However, intoxication also can be dysphoric and anxiogenic, leading to social withdrawal, panic, and even paranoia. These latter effects are more common in inexperienced users. Physiological symptoms of intoxication are well established and include increased appetite, tachycardia and tachypnea, elevated blood pressure or orthostasis, ocular erythema, and dry mouth. Less common physical symptoms of intoxication include nystagmus, ataxia, and slurred speech.

Box 8–1 contains DSM-5 criteria for cannabis intoxication (American Psychiatric Association 2013).

Box 8–1. Diagnostic Criteria for Cannabis Intoxication

A. Recent use of cannabis.

B. Clinically significant problematic behavioral or psychological changes (e.g., impaired motor coordination, euphoria, anxiety, sensation of slowed time, impaired judgment, social withdrawal) that developed during, or shortly after, cannabis use.

C. Two (or more) of the following signs or symptoms developing within 2 hours of cannabis use:

1. Conjunctival injection.
2. Increased appetite.
3. Dry mouth.
4. Tachycardia.

D. The signs or symptoms are not attributable to another medical condition and are not better explained by another mental disorder, including intoxication with another substance.

Specify if:
   With perceptual disturbances

What to Do About Intoxication

Management of cannabis intoxication is supportive and varies by the age of the user and the severity of intoxication.

Cannabis intoxication can be fatal in children when it causes hyperkinesis, seizures, or coma. Central nervous system depression in the child should be treated with supportive care and respiratory support if needed. Seizures should be treated with benzodiazepines.

In adolescents and adults, intoxication can range from mild to severe. Mild intoxication is marked by anxiety and dysphoria that can be managed with environmental interventions that decrease stimulation and benzodiazepines if needed. Severe intoxication with cannabis is rare, and management of such episodes is discussed in the section "Synthetic Cannabinoids" later in this chapter.

How to Recognize Withdrawal

Cannabis withdrawal can be uncomfortable and distressing, but it is not life-threatening. THC redistributes into adipose tissues, extending the elimination half-life. This property can reduce the severity of withdrawal symptoms but also can extend their duration. Typically, the onset of withdrawal is within 24 hours after cessation of cannabis use, peaks within 1 week, and lasts 1–2 weeks. Some symptoms of withdrawal can persist for weeks and may contribute to relapse.

Common symptoms of withdrawal:

- Fatigue or hypersomnia
- Yawning
- Psychomotor retardation
- Anxiety, dysphoria, and irritability
- Anorexia and weight loss
- Strange dreams

Persistent symptoms of withdrawal:

- Sleep disturbance, typically insomnia
- Irritability
- Physical tension

Box 8–2 contains DSM-5 criteria for cannabis withdrawal.

Box 8–2.   Diagnostic Criteria for Cannabis Withdrawal

A. Cessation of cannabis use that has been heavy and prolonged (i.e., usually daily or almost daily use over a period of at least a few months).
B. Three (or more) of the following signs and symptoms develop within approximately 1 week after Criterion A:
   1. Irritability, anger, or aggression.
   2. Nervousness or anxiety.
   3. Sleep difficulty (e.g., insomnia, disturbing dreams).
   4. Decreased appetite or weight loss.
   5. Restlessness.
   6. Depressed mood.
   7. At least one of the following physical symptoms causing significant discomfort: abdominal pain, shakiness/tremors, sweating, fever, chills, or headache.

C. The signs or symptoms in Criterion B cause clinically significant distress or impairment in social, occupational, or other important areas of functioning.

D. The signs or symptoms are not attributable to another medical condition and are not better explained by another mental disorder, including intoxication or withdrawal from another substance.

What to Do About Withdrawal

Withdrawal from cannabis is not life-threatening, and symptoms should be managed according to the goals of treatment. Little clinical evidence indicates that the treatment of withdrawal symptoms reduces the likelihood of relapse, but there is a theoretical correlation, and the treatment of withdrawal symptoms can reduce a patient's discomfort. In one study, more than a quarter of cannabis users reported using cannabis to relieve or avoid withdrawal symptoms (Copersino et al. 2006). In the section "What to Do About Addiction" later in this chapter, medications that can help attenuate withdrawal symptoms are discussed.

How to Recognize Addiction

A patient who meets DSM-5 criteria for cannabis use disorder (Box 8–3) may report continued use of cannabis despite subjective distress or adverse personal consequences. He or she also may present with evidence of impairment in social and occupational functioning that he or she has not linked to the use of cannabis. Cannabis use has been associated with higher rates of school dropout, crime, and unemployment. Additional signs of addiction are shown in the DSM-5 criteria for cannabis use disorder.

Box 8–3. Diagnostic Criteria for Cannabis Use Disorder

A. A problematic pattern of cannabis use leading to clinically significant impairment or distress, as manifested by at least two of the following, occurring within a 12-month period:

   1. Cannabis is often taken in larger amounts or over a longer period than was intended.

   2. There is a persistent desire or unsuccessful efforts to cut down or control cannabis use.

3. A great deal of time is spent in activities necessary to obtain cannabis, use cannabis, or recover from its effects.
4. Craving, or a strong desire or urge to use cannabis.
5. Recurrent cannabis use resulting in a failure to fulfill major role obligations at work, school, or home.
6. Continued cannabis use despite having persistent or recurrent social or interpersonal problems caused or exacerbated by the effects of cannabis.
7. Important social, occupational, or recreational activities are given up or reduced because of cannabis use.
8. Recurrent cannabis use in situations in which it is physically hazardous.
9. Cannabis use is continued despite knowledge of having a persistent or recurrent physical or psychological problem that is likely to have been caused or exacerbated by cannabis.
10. Tolerance, as defined by either of the following:
    a. A need for markedly increased amounts of cannabis to achieve intoxication or desired effect.
    b. Markedly diminished effect with continued use of the same amount of cannabis.
11. Withdrawal, as manifested by either of the following:
    a. The characteristic withdrawal syndrome for cannabis (refer to Criteria A and B of the criteria set for cannabis withdrawal).
    b. Cannabis (or a closely related substance) is taken to relieve or avoid withdrawal symptoms.

Specify if:
In early remission
In sustained remission

Specify if:
In a controlled environment

Specify current severity:
Mild: Presence of 2–3 symptoms.
Moderate: Presence of 4–5 symptoms.
Severe: Presence of 6 or more symptoms.

Cannabis is most commonly used by persons ages 18–25 and is rarely used before age 13. Among those who use cannabis, the risk for cannabis use disorder has been found to be highest in adolescents ages 17–18 years. Beyond age 30, the risk of developing cannabis use disorder is minimal. Overall, it is estimated that fewer than 10% of individuals who try cannabis will ever meet the clinical criteria for dependence, whereas of those who try tobacco and alcohol, 32% and 15%, respectively, will eventually meet the clinical criteria for dependence (Joy et al. 1999; Substance Abuse and Mental Health Services Administration Center for Behavioral Health Statistics and Quality 2014).

When assessing a patient, clinicians should consider risk factors to help guide diagnosis. There is a heritable genetic risk for cannabis use disorder. Population-based predictors include the comorbid use of other drugs and the use of cannabis by peers or family members. Men are more likely than women to develop cannabis use disorder. Race and ethnicity have not been shown to be significantly associated with the development of cannabis use disorder. Residence in an urban or rural setting and income level also are not associated with increased risk for the development of cannabis use disorder.

What to Do About Addiction

The provider usually will treat cannabis use disorder in the outpatient setting, with residential or inpatient treatment limited to those with other comorbid substance use disorders or psychiatric disorders necessitating a more restrictive setting. Treatment should consist of a combination of psychosocial therapy, pharmacotherapy, and lifestyle interventions.

PSYCHOTHERAPY

In general, psychosocial treatments have been shown to produce modest reductions in use and little to no effect on abstinence rates. However, interventions will be most effective if they focus on education about the potential consequences of cannabis use, the enhancement of motivation to reduce cannabis use or achieve abstinence, and the alteration of reinforcement contingencies. Other targets of psychosocial interventions include enhancing the management of painful affects while improving social supports and social functioning.

For adults, motivational enhancement therapy, individual and group cognitive-behavioral therapy (CBT), and contingency management are effective when used alone or in combination. Peer support groups such as Marijuana Anonymous are available to those with cannabis use disorder, but their efficacy has not been rigorously studied. Adolescents also benefit from CBT and contingency management, but family-based treatments are the most successful.

PHARMACOTHERAPY

Unfortunately, little evidence indicates that medication can reduce cannabis use or improve outcomes in cannabis use disorder. Most medication treatment focuses on the reduction of symptoms associated with early abstinence and protracted abstinence syndromes.

N-ACETYLCYSTEINE

N-Acetylcysteine (NAC) is a derivative of the amino acid cysteine that modulates glutamate and dopamine transmission. It is the most well-supported treatment for cannabis use disorder, with one randomized controlled trial showing that it reduced the likelihood of positive urine toxicology for THC in comparison to treatment with placebo (Gray et al. 2012). The typical dose for NAC is 1,200 mg orally twice a day. It is a relatively safe medication that the patient can purchase over the counter.

ANTICONVULSANTS

One randomized controlled clinical trial of CBT and valproic acid treatment versus CBT and placebo found no clinically significant improvements in outcomes. Gabapentin was shown to reduce cannabis use by self-report and as evidenced by urine toxicology. It was also shown to reduce withdrawal symptoms. However, one limitation was high dropout rates.

ANTIDEPRESSANTS

Nefazodone and bupropion had effects similar to those of placebo when combined with individual counseling, but their trials also had high dropout rates.

BUSPIRONE

Studies of buspirone have been nonsignificant.

CANNABINOID AGONISTS

Rimonabant is a CB_1 partial agonist that has been shown to blunt the subjective effects of smoked cannabis by 40%, but this result has not been replicated (Huestis et al. 2001). It also failed to achieve approval in the United States as a weight loss drug because of psychiatric adverse events. Dronabinol is a CB_1 agonist that has been shown to reduce symptoms of withdrawal when compared with placebo. However, it has not been shown to reduce laboratory models of relapse or cannabis self-administration.

PARASYMPATHOMIMETICS

Lofexidine is an α_2 agonist that may reduce the adrenergic symptoms common to withdrawal syndromes from many substances. It is unclear at this point whether lofexidine would reduce the likelihood of relapse in comparison to placebo. Clonidine, another α_2 agonist, has been shown to blunt signs of withdrawal in animal studies.

ZOLPIDEM

Zolpidem has been shown to attenuate abstinence-induced sleep disturbance. Theoretically, this could reduce the likelihood of relapse to cannabis use, but no definitive evidence supports this effect.

RECOMMENDATIONS

Psychotherapeutic treatment should combine contingency management with CBT or motivational enhancement therapy, depending on the patient's stage of change. The patient also should be offered a referral to a peer group. Children and adolescents especially should have family therapy as a mainstay of treatment. Behavioral modification that has been shown to be helpful in the treatment of other substance use disorders should be considered; for example, yoga has some support in the treatment of cannabis use disorder. The only medication with evidence of reducing cannabis use is NAC (1,200 mg orally twice a day). Dronabinol for withdrawal in general or medications to target specific symptoms of withdrawal such as short-term zolpidem for insomnia also may be tried. Comorbid psychiatric disorders should be treated in concert with cannabis use disorder.

Special Issues With Psychiatric Comorbidities

Cannabis use has been associated with impaired psychological functioning, including poorer life satisfaction, higher rates of depression, anxiety disorders, suicide attempts, and conduct disorder. Cannabis use disorder is associated with comorbid psychiatric disorders: an estimated 24% of individuals with cannabis use disorder have an anxiety disorder, 13% have bipolar I disorder, and 11% have major depressive disorder (Ries et al. 2014). Cannabis use also has been identified as a risk factor for earlier-onset schizophrenia and a predictor of worse outcomes when comorbid with schizophrenia. In general, individuals with a mental illness and comorbid cannabis use disorder have been shown to be less likely to adhere to treatment, and they have been shown to use more mental health treatment resources. Although research has not established a causal relation between cannabis use and mental illness, the association with worse outcomes requires attention during treatment.

Cannabis use also has been associated with impaired cognitive performance. This association has biological plausibility because cannabinoid receptors are located in areas associated with memory and attention. In acute intoxication, animal studies have shown that intoxication impairs focused and divided attention, short-term and episodic memory, complex cognitive processing, and motor ability. All these impairments have been shown to moderate with tolerance. In chronic use, studies have suggested problems with filtering out complex irrelevant information, mental flexibility, working memory, learning, and sustained attention, with worse long-term cognitive effects in smokers who initiate cannabis use at a younger age (Ries et al. 2014).

Cannabis use has been shown to lead to selective cognitive impairments, but the magnitude and functional significance of these impairments are unclear. Cannabis may reduce the ability of intoxicated persons to react to emergent situations while driving; however, it also has been associated with reduced risk-taking behavior and fatal accidents. Cannabis use has been associated with lower grade point average, negative attitudes toward school, and truancy; but in many studies that controlled for confounding factors, these associations were attenuated. A review of 19 studies (Segev and Lev-Ran 2012) examined cognitive effects of cannabis on schizophrenia by comparing patients with schizophrenia who smoked cannabis with those who did not; the review found that 11 studies actually reported better cognitive function in patients using cannabis, 5 found minimal or no differences, and 3 found poorer functioning. "Amotivational symptoms" are described in some reviews of cannabis use, but other studies have found no effect of cannabis use on motivation.

Cannabis use disorder is associated with comorbid use of other substances. Cannabis often has been referred to as a gateway drug. In fact, most people who use cannabis will not progress to use other drugs. However, the presence of comorbid use with other substances signals to the practitioner the potential for worse outcomes.

Special Issues With Medical Comorbidities

The following discussion highlights medical conditions that can be exacerbated by both acute and chronic cannabis use, especially when smoked (Ries et al. 2014). However, it should be noted that research is ongoing into possible therapeutic applications of cannabinoids.

RESPIRATORY

Cannabis smoke actually has been shown to contain a higher density of tar and a greater number of carcinogens than tobacco smoke. However, the cannabis user tends to smoke less than the tobacco user does, which may be the reason that chronic cannabis use has not been found to be associated with a reduction in pulmonary function. However, cannabis users do have higher rates of disorders associated with chronic airway inflammation, such as bronchitis. In the acute setting, cannabis smoke can exacerbate asthma and has rarely been implicated in the development of pneumomediastinum and pneumothorax.

ONCOLOGICAL

Cannabis may be associated with increased risk of cancer on the basis of molecular and cellular evidence that smoking cannabis could cause neoplastic changes. However, clinical research is inconclusive because studies have tended to be underpowered or confounded by the presence of comorbid tobacco use.

CARDIOVASCULAR

Cannabis intoxication is associated with mild tachycardia, which is likely clinically insignificant in most patients. Patients with cardiovascular disease may be more at risk from these effects, and cannabis intoxication rarely has been associated with myocardial infarction. In the elderly, orthostasis in the setting of cannabis intoxication can lead to presyncopal falls and injuries.

HEPATIC

Cannabis use has been linked to steatosis and so may be deleterious for chronic users who also have liver disease.

IMMUNOLOGICAL

The effects of cannabis use on CB_2 receptors and their role in immune response are little understood at this time. However, there is interest in regard to possible therapeutic indications.

ENDOCRINE

Cannabinoids can alter hormone levels through their interaction with the pituitary gland, inhibiting release of luteinizing hormone, growth hormone, and prolactin. Cannabinoids have been shown to affect thyroid hormone release in animals but not in humans. The clinical significance of these effects is unclear, although cannabis is thought to disrupt the female reproductive system and to induce galactorrhea.

Synthetic Cannabinoids

Medical research on cannabis was banned in the United States in the 1970s, and as a result, synthetic cannabinoids were first created as legal substrates to be used only in scientific research; they were never intended for human consumption (Sacco and Finklea 2014). Despite the initial intention of synthetic cannabinoids for scientific research, recreational abuse has become prevalent.

In the United States, synthetic cannabinoids are most commonly used by young men in their 20s and 30s, but they are also used by adolescents. In 2012, 11% of adolescents in twelfth grade were identified as smoking synthetic cannabinoids; this number dropped to 5% in 2015 (National Institute on Drug Abuse 2015). Although these compounds have physiological effects similar to those of cannabis, they have a greater potential to cause neuropsychiatric side effects, including delirium, psychosis, and hallucinations, as well as life-threatening toxic effects, including seizures and severe agitation.

Abuse of synthetic cannabinoids has progressed quickly, in part because of their availability as legal, uncontrolled substances sold commercially in tobacco shops. In reaction to high rates of emergency department visits associated with synthetic cannabinoid use, the synthetic cannabinoids are now designated as Schedule I drugs. However, their use remains prevalent as new synthetic cannabinoids find their way to store shelves before they are identified and rescheduled. Thus, despite efforts to restrict their distribution, the continued development of synthetic compounds effectively renews the supply of synthetic cannabinoids for public consumption.

PHARMACOLOGY

Synthetic cannabinoids are analogues of naturally occurring chemicals in the cannabis plant, such as THC, cannabidiol, and cannabinol. They are synthesized to have a much higher potency than their analogues found in marijuana. They can be both partial and full agonists at the cannabinoid receptors and have different pharmacokinetics. Unlike cannabis, they can be ingested and insufflated in their pure form and exist without the balance of other cannabinoid active substances found in marijuana.

As a group, their chemical properties and pharmacokinetics vary. Clinical manifestations typically occur soon after inhalation or intranasal use and can last several hours to days.

Urine tests are available for synthetic cannabinoids, but the increasing variety of compounds, the relatively poor availability of tests, and the lack of rapid tests render urine toxicology screening for synthetic cannabinoids clinically irrelevant.

HOW TO RECOGNIZE INTOXICATION

Synthetic cannabinoids bind to the same receptors as cannabis and produce similar clinical manifestations. Therefore, DSM-5 criteria for cannabis use disorder, cannabis intoxication, and cannabis withdrawal are applicable to individuals using synthetic cannabinoids (American Psychiatric Association 2013). However, symptoms can be more severe than cannabis and in some cases lethal.

Persons with synthetic cannabinoid intoxication usually present to the emergency department with symptoms of tachycardia, agitation, and vomiting. However, hallucinations, dystonia, dysarthria, short-term memory deficits, and paranoia can be present. Rarely, patients with synthetic cannabinoid intoxication may present with severe psychomotor agitation, psychotic symptoms, delirium, or seizures. Psychomotor agitation and seizures can be life-threatening, resulting in hyperthermia and rhabdomyolysis progressing to acute kidney injury. There have also been case reports of chest pain and myocardial infarction in adolescents and young adults presenting to the emergency department with synthetic cannabinoid intoxication.

WHAT TO DO ABOUT INTOXICATION

As in cannabis intoxication, the treatment of synthetic cannabinoid intoxication is supportive. For mild to moderate intoxication, symptoms may be limited to anxiety, paranoia, and dysphoria. Treatment should consist of creating a nonthreatening, minimally stimulating environment with benzodiazepine treatment if needed.

For severe intoxication, management decisions are based on the presenting symptoms. Agitation and psychosis should be treated primarily with environmental interventions and secondarily by pharmaceutical treatment if needed for safety. Benzodiazepine treatment is the first-line pharmacotherapy for synthetic cannabinoid–related agitation and hyperthermia.

Rhabdomyolysis may occur if a patient experiences severe agitation, hyperthermia, seizures, and muscle rigidity. In this setting, the goal of treatment is adequate hydration with intravenous fluids to reduce the likelihood of acute renal failure. Benzodiazepines can be used if the patient is experiencing seizures.

Dystonic reactions should be treated with short-acting benzodiazepines.

KEY POINTS

Cannabinoids have been shown to be addictive, produce tolerance, and induce a withdrawal syndrome that can contribute to relapse. Maladaptive patterns of cannabis use can have social, occupational, medical, and psychiatric consequences.

Treatment of cannabis use disorder should combine psychotherapeutic approaches—including motivational enhancement therapy, cognitive-behavioral therapy, contingency management, and peer support groups—with *N*-acetylcysteine 1,200 mg orally twice a day, and other medications that may help blunt symptoms of withdrawal.

Recent changes in cannabis policy may increase the availability of the drug but also may increase availability of treatment while reducing the social consequences of high rates of imprisonment.

Synthetic cannabinoids are relatively new drugs of abuse that are similar to cannabis, but because of higher potency and selective purity, they can cause lethal physiological and disturbing psychiatric and behavioral symptoms.

References

American Psychiatric Association: Diagnostic and Statistical Manual of Mental Disorders, 5th Edition. Arlington, VA, American Psychiatric Association, 2013

Copersino ML, Boyd SJ, Tashkin DP, et al: Cannabis withdrawal among non-treatment-seeking adult cannabis users. Am J Addict 15(1):8–14, 2006 16449088

Gray KM, Carpenter MJ, Baker NL, et al: A double-blind randomized controlled trial of N-acetylcysteine in cannabis-dependent adolescents. Am J Psychiatry 169(8):805–812, 2012 22706327

Huestis MA, Gorelick DA, Heishman SJ, et al: Blockade of effects of smoked marijuana by the CB1-selective cannabinoid receptor antagonist SR141716. Arch Gen Psychiatry 58(4):322–328, 2001 11296091

Joy JE, Watson SJ Jr, Benson JA (eds): Marijuana and Medicine: Assessing the Science Base. Washington, DC, National Academy Press, 1999

National Institute on Drug Abuse: Monitoring the Future Survey, Overview of Findings 2015, December 2015. Available at: http://www.drugabuse.gov/related-topics/trends-statistics/monitoring-future/monitoring-future-survey-overview-findings-2015. Accessed March 2, 2016.

Ries RK, Fiellin DA, Miller SC, et al (eds): The ASAM Principles of Addiction Medicine, 5th Edition. Philadelphia, PA, Lippincott Williams & Wilkins, 2014

Ross S, Peselow E: The neurobiology of addictive disorders. Clin Neuropharmacol 32(5):269–276, 2009 19834992

Sacco LN, Finklea K: Synthetic Drugs: Overview and Issues for Congress. Washington, DC, Congressional Research Service, August 15, 2014. Available at: http://www.fas.org/sgp/crs/misc/R42066.pdf. Accessed December 22, 2015.

Segev A, Lev-Ran S: Neurocognitive functioning and cannabis use in schizophrenia. Curr Pharm Des 18(32):4999–5007, 2012 22716156

Substance Abuse and Mental Health Services Administration Center for Behavioral Health Statistics and Quality: Results From the 2013 National Survey on Drug Use and Health: Summary of National Findings. Rockville, MD, U.S. Department of Health and Human Services, 2014. Available at: http://www.samhsa.gov/data/sites/default/files/NSDUHresultsPDFWHTML2013/Web/NSDUHresults2013.pdf. Accessed December 22, 2015.

CHAPTER 9

Hallucinogens and Dissociative Drugs

C. ALEXANDER PALEOS, M.D.

CLASSIC (serotonergic) hallucinogens, atypical hallucinogens, and dissociative drugs represent a wide range of substances with different pharmacological profiles, addictive liability, and lethality with use. All of these agents can be the source of specific diagnoses of hallucinogen-related substance disorders described in DSM-5 criteria (American Psychiatric Association 2013)—although certain agents would rarely result in a syndrome requiring diagnosis, as discussed later in this chapter. Table 9–1 contains a list of street names for some of these drugs.

Overview

CLASSIC (SEROTONERGIC) HALLUCINOGENS

The following are the **classic (serotonergic) hallucinogens:**

- Lysergic acid diethylamide (LSD)
- Psilocybin
- Mescaline
- *N,N*-dimethyltryptamine (DMT)

The classic hallucinogens are clearly distinct from drugs with true addictive liability—such as heroin, cocaine, and alcohol. This is neither to dismiss nor to minimize the great harm these substances can and do cause when used irresponsibly, but more than 50 years of epidemiological data fail to establish a link between the classic hallucinogens and the development of dependence syndromes. Users, who tend to be in their adolescence and early adulthood, do not experience withdrawal

TABLE 9–1. Street names for selected hallucinogens and dissociative drugs

Drug name	Street names
Lysergic acid diethylamide (LSD)	Acid, Blotter, Microdots, Window panes
Psilocybin	Magic mushrooms, Shrooms
3,4-Methylenedioxy-methamphetamine (MDMA)	Ecstasy, Molly, Adam, Beans, E, X, Thizz, Rolls
2-(4-iodo-2,5-dimethoxy-phenyl)-N-[(2-methoxy-phenyl)methyl]ethana-mine (2C-I-NBOMe/ 25I-NBOMe)	N-Bomb, Smiles, 25I, Wizard
2,5-dimethoxy-4-n-propylthiophenethyl-amine (2C-T-7)	T7, Blue Mystic
2,5-dimethoxy-4-ethyl-phenethylamine (2C-E)	Europa
Salvia/Salvinorin A	Sally D, Magic mint, Maria Pastora, Diviner's sage
Phencyclidine (PCP)	Angel dust, Dust, Hog, Ozone, Horse tranquilizer, Wack, Crystal, Sherms; Embalming fluid (liquid form); Dippers/ Supergrass/Love boat (when combined with cannabis)
Ketamine	K, Special K, Vitamin K, Cat valium, Kit kat
Dextromethorphan (DXM)	Dex, Robo, Tussin, Triple C, Skittles, Red hots

symptoms or cravings and do not engage in compulsive drug-seeking behaviors, and the vast majority spontaneously reduce or stop their use over time. Thus, the National Institute on Drug Abuse (NIDA) does not categorize hallucinogens as drugs of "addiction," even though they are classified as drugs of abuse (Schedule I) and criminalized to the furthest extent possible both in the United States and abroad.

Under the influence of these substances, users experience profound disturbances of perception, as the term *hallucinogen* implies. However, at typical psychoactive doses, what occur are not frank hallucinations but perceptual alterations of genuine sensory input, more correctly termed *illusions*. The term *hallucinogen* furthermore fails to convey the profound changes in cognition and emotional responsiveness that these substances also invariably induce. Despite their powerful psychological effects, the classic hallucinogens are, physiologically, remarkably benign, and none are known to be lethal in overdose.

However, the health dangers posed by irresponsible use of these substances provide ample justification for their being controlled. When taken in the absence of appropriate safeguards, particularly at high doses and under adverse circumstances, hallucinogens are likely to precipitate a "bad trip," a harrowing psychological experience characterized by anxiety, paranoia, and/or agitation; these symptoms are the most likely to attract medical attention. Despite these agents' benign physiological profile, accidental deaths and suicides certainly do occur under their judgment-impairing influence and are the greatest danger these substances pose when used recreationally. Almost as dire are the potential consequences for someone with a biological predisposition to psychotic illness, because the psychiatric sequelae for such individuals can be permanently disabling.

The associated contextual factors of *set* (the mind-set of the person ingesting the substance) and *setting* (the social and environmental context in which the ingestion takes place) are crucial to the ensuing psychological effects of any classic hallucinogen, which are always powerful but, depending on these factors, can vary from profoundly beneficial to catastrophic. For example, LSD was first synthesized in a pharmaceutical lab and was responsibly used in legitimate research settings for decades before it was diverted to the streets in the 1960s. Its use then quickly became indiscriminate, with extremely adverse consequences the all-too-frequent result. Naturally occurring hallucinogens, such as psilocybin, mescaline, and DMT, were used by indigenous peoples for at least 6,000 years as ritual sacraments, before their conversion into drugs of abuse.

Recent years have seen the careful resurgence of a second wave of federally approved clinical research on serotonergic hallucinogens, principally psilocybin. Studies that use psilocybin-assisted motivational enhancement therapy for the treatment of nicotine dependence and alcoholism are currently under way, and the preliminary results for these indications appear to be promising. Psilocybin is also being investigated in a multisite Phase III clinical trial of psychotherapy for cancer-related anxiety and depression.

ATYPICAL HALLUCINOGENS

The following substances are **atypical hallucinogens:**

- 3,4-Methylenedioxymethamphetamine (MDMA)
- Substituted phenethylamines ("designer drugs")
- Salvinorin A (*Salvia*)

MDMA was initially patented by Merck Pharmaceuticals in 1914 and was used as an adjunctive tool for insight-oriented therapy (Holland 2001). It was highly valued for its properties as an entactogen (facilitating touch with internal states), which were believed to permit patients to explore and integrate severe psychological trauma that would otherwise be too emotionally painful to access in a safe or effective way. A boom of recreational MDMA use resulted in its classification as Schedule I, which contributed to its widespread underground use in the 1990s within the rave culture of the United Kingdom and later the United States, where it became known as "Ecstasy" or "Molly." It remains a popular drug of abuse; in 2011, it was second only to phencyclidine (PCP) as a cause of emergency department visits in the United States (Table 9–2). In contrast to the classic hallucinogens, it can be lethal in overdose and can contribute to other potentially fatal complications such as heatstroke and hyponatremia.

The so-called designer drugs comprise an increasingly large number of synthetic pharmaceuticals that are in most cases structurally similar to existing controlled substances. These include synthetic cannabinoids (see Chapter 8, "Cannabis"), synthetic cathinones (see Chapter 12, "Stimulants"), and the substituted phenethylamines. Hundreds are avail-

TABLE 9–2. Demographics for emergency department visits in 2011, by drug of abuse

Drug[a]	Total visits	% of emergency department drug visits[b]	Male	Female	Younger than 21	21 and older	White	Black	Hispanic
Phencyclidine (PCP)	75,538	6.1	51,906	23,598	5,699	69,774	23,485	43,599	3,677
3,4-Methylenedioxy-methamphetamine (MDMA)	22,498	1.8	15,612	6,886	10,176	12,316	11,421	4,352	3,089
Miscellaneous hallucinogens	8,043	0.6	6,758	1,285	4,665	3,374	5,775	296	NR
Lysergic acid diethylamide (LSD)	4,819	0.4	4,045	773	2,347	2,471	3,393	NR	NR
Ketamine	1,550	0.1	1,124	NR	NR	954	1,261	NR	NR

TABLE 9–2. Demographics for emergency department visits in 2011, by drug of abuse *(continued)*

Drug[a]	Total visits	% of emergency department visits[b]	Male	Female	Younger than 21	21 and older	White	Black	Hispanic
Antitussives (including dextromethorphan)	1,515	0.1	1,454	NR	1,101	NR	917	NR	NR

Note. NR=data not reported.

[a]No data were reported for ethnicities other than white, black, or Hispanic for any of the substances listed.

[b]Total emergency department drug visits excludes patients age 21 and older presenting with alcohol involvement only.

Source. Adapted from Drug Abuse Warning Network: National Estimates of Emergency Department Visits, 2004–2011. Available at: http://www.samhsa.gov/data/emergency-department-data-dawn/reports. Accessed February 28, 2015.

able for purchase on the Internet, and their sellers hope to exploit their novelty to circumvent drug laws. Unfortunately, these substances are frequently more potent and more toxic than their target analogues, and the newer they are, the less is known about their safety. Among the newest and most problematic is 2-(4-iodo-2,5-dimethoxyphenyl)-*N*-[(2-methoxyphenyl)methyl]ethanamine, also known as 2C-I-NBOMe or 25I-NBOMe and on the street as "N-Bomb." Its effects are reportedly both hallucinogenic and entactogenic, and its potency approaches that of LSD, with effective doses in the microgram range. Unlike LSD, however, it can be lethal in overdose, and several fatalities have been reported since 2012. Overdose deaths also have occurred with 2C-T-7 (2,5-dimethoxy-4-*n*-propylthiophenethylamine), 2C-E (2,5-dimethoxy-4-ethylphenethylamine), and 3C-bromo-dragonfly (1-(8-bromo-benzo[1,2-b;4,5-b']difuran-4-yl)-2-aminopropane).

Salvia divinorum, or "diviner's sage," is an herb in the mint family native to southern Mexico, where it has been used by indigenous shamans and healers for centuries. In this context, *Salvia* is ingested orally, either by chewing the leaves or by drinking a juice extracted from them. In industrialized nations where *Salvia* is abused, it is almost always smoked, which results in a much more intense, albeit considerably briefer, hallucinatory and dissociative effect. NIDA reported that *Salvia* had overtaken LSD and PCP as the most commonly abused hallucinogenic drug in the United States from 2009 to 2013 among high school seniors (Johnston et al. 2015; National Institute on Drug Abuse 2015), although *Salvia* is not associated with addiction syndromes. (In 2014, its use declined and was surpassed by LSD, although use of both substances decreased.) The abuse of *Salvia* is at least partly attributable to its availability and legal status; at present, *Salvia* is not federally controlled, but most states have now passed laws to criminalize it. Street names include "magic mint" and "Sally D."

DISSOCIATIVE DRUGS

The following substances are **dissociative drugs:**

- Phencyclidine (PCP)
- Ketamine
- Dextromethorphan (DXM)

Originally an anesthetic removed from the market because of its postoperative effects, PCP arrived on the street in the late

1960s and became one of the most frequently abused drugs by the late 1970s. Since the 1980s, its use has declined considerably, although use has increased in recent years. In its crystalline form, PCP is most often smoked but can be snorted or taken orally. It can also be obtained in a liquid form referred to as "embalming fluid," with which cannabis or tobacco cigarettes are coated to produce "dippers." Among the drugs in this chapter, it is by far the most likely to precipitate a visit to an emergency department, accounting for more visits than all other hallucinogens and dissociative drugs combined (see Table 9–2).

Ketamine was first synthesized as a derivative of PCP in 1962 and has been used as a surgical anesthetic and procedural sedative since 1970, an indication for which it continues to be widely used. It has received intense scrutiny from psychiatric researchers because of the discovery of its efficacy as a rapid-acting antidepressant at subanesthetic doses. Beginning in the mid-1980s, it gained popularity as a "club drug," and its recreational use continues unabated to the present day. Street names include "Special K" or simply "K" (note that "K2" is the name of a synthetic cannabinoid and does not refer to ketamine). Most often, it is obtained in its powdered form and snorted in "bumps"; as a liquid or powder, it can also be injected, smoked, or mixed into drinks and ingested orally. Because it is colorless and odorless, the latter method has been implicated in cases of drug-facilitated sexual assault, particularly on college campuses.

DXM is an antitussive medication available in more than 120 over-the-counter formulations. At low doses, it is safe and effective as a cough suppressant, but at higher doses, it induces effects similar to those of PCP and ketamine. For many years, it was sold only as a syrup with a taste that was designed to discourage large-volume ingestions, but more recently, it has become available in gel-tab form, with a candy-like appearance, lending itself to the street name "Skittles" and to abuse by adolescents; its abuse has thus become increasingly prevalent, particularly among this age group.

Pharmacology

CLASSIC (SEROTONERGIC) HALLUCINOGENS

The classic hallucinogens can be divided into two subcategories: 1) the tryptamines, which structurally resemble serotonin and include psilocybin, DMT, and LSD; and 2) the phenethylamines, such as mescaline, which are structurally similar to norepinephrine. As their name implies, the activity of all serotonergic hallucinogens is thought to be primarily mediated by the serotonin neurotransmitter system (Table 9–3). Specifically, serotonin type 2A (5-HT_{2A}) receptor agonism is considered central to their effects, although activity at 5-HT_{2C} and 5-HT_{1A} receptors is also likely to play a role. LSD has a more complex structure and binding profile than the other tryptamines, with only partial agonism at 5-$HT_{1A/2A}$ receptors and agonist activity at dopamine type 2 (D_2) receptor and α-adrenergic receptors. How any of these molecular interactions translate into the profound subjective effects of the classic hallucinogens remains incompletely understood but seems to involve modulation of the neural circuitry responsible for sensory gating and regulation of the boundaries of self-awareness.

The classic hallucinogens, with the exception of DMT, induce a rapid form of tolerance known as *tachyphylaxis*, likely mediated by potent downregulation of the 5-HT_{2A} receptor. Daily administration of LSD, for example, results in nearly complete loss of activity by the fourth day despite escalations in dose, an effect that results in cross-tolerance to psilocybin and mescaline as well (Nichols 2004).

Importantly, the classic hallucinogens are characterized by an absence of dopamine upregulation in the mesolimbic pathway, which renders them essentially incapable of producing physiological dependence syndromes.

ATYPICAL HALLUCINOGENS

In contrast to the classic hallucinogens, MDMA has very weak affinity for the 5-HT_{2A} receptor. Its mechanism is more similar to that of methamphetamine, as it induces presynaptic release of serotonin, dopamine, and norepinephrine (Table 9–4). Unlike methamphetamine, however, MDMA's effects are much more pronounced for serotonin than for dopamine. MDMA also acts as a serotonin reuptake inhibitor, further amplifying synaptic concentrations of serotonin. Nonetheless, its effect on mesolimbic dopamine levels is sufficient to induce increased self-administration in animal models, and in humans its use can lead to an addiction syndrome.

The pharmacology of the substituted phenethylamines is less well characterized, although it is known that they bind to 5-HT_2 receptors, acting as agonists or antagonists depending on the subtype.

TABLE 9–3. Pharmacological profiles of selected classic hallucinogens

	Lysergic acid diethylamide (LSD)	Psilocybin	*N,N*-dimethyltryptamine (DMT)	Mescaline
Mechanism of action	5-HT$_{1A/2A}$ partial agonism	5-HT$_{1A/2A}$ agonism	5-HT$_{1A/2A}$ agonism	5-HT$_{1A/2A}$ agonism
Psychoactive dosing range	25–400 µg	0.25–5 g (dried mushrooms)	10–60 mg	10–40 g (dried peyote buttons)
Typical route(s) of ingestion	Oral	Oral	Smoked	Oral
Time to onset	20–60 min	15–60 min	15–60 s	1–2 h
Approximate time to peak effect	90 min	90 min	90 s	3 h
Duration of effect	6–11 h	4–7 h	6–20 min	5–8 h

Note. 5-HT$_{1A/2A}$ = serotonin type 1A/2A receptor.

Salvinorin A is a diterpene alkaloid and a κ opioid receptor agonist. It is also the most potent naturally occurring hallucinogen, with 20 times the potency of psilocybin and about half that of LSD. Unique among hallucinogenic substances, it exerts its effects completely independently of the serotonin system. With regard to the opioid system, its binding is highly selective for κ receptors, showing no activity at μ or δ receptors.

DISSOCIATIVE DRUGS

PCP and ketamine are arylcyclohexylamines that act as noncompetitive antagonists of the *N*-methyl-D-aspartate (NMDA) glutamate receptor (Table 9–5). Their dissociative effects are thought to be mediated by an uncoupling of the limbic and thalamoneocortical systems. Ketamine also binds to μ opioid receptors, which may contribute to its analgesic effects. PCP and ketamine are unique among anesthetic agents in that they stimulate rather than suppress the sympathetic nervous system, an effect likely mediated by α-adrenergic agonism.

DXM is the dextrorotatory stereoisomer of levomethorphan, a codeine analogue and opioid agonist. Because of this difference in stereochemistry, DXM has very little affinity for μ or δ opioid receptors. At the recommended therapeutic dosage, its antitussive effects are mediated by σ receptors. At the high doses taken recreationally, DXM antagonizes NMDA receptors, with effects similar to those of ketamine.

TOXICOLOGY

Of the substances in this chapter, PCP is the only one commonly included in standard urine drug screens. Nevertheless, urine drug screens should be universally performed if hallucinogen or dissociative drug intoxication is suspected because of the high incidence of polysubstance abuse in these users. Of note, MDMA cross-reacts and tests positive with standard urine amphetamine assays of sufficient sensitivity (500 ng/mL or lower); it is detectable for 1–3 days with single use and 3–5 days with heavy use. PCP remains detectable in urine for approximately 3–7 days after a single ingestion, but habitual users may test positive for up to 30 days because of its high lipid solubility. Both ketamine and DXM can cross-react (albeit unreliably) to yield false-positive PCP assays, which may provide useful information if abuse of these substances is suspected.

TABLE 9-4. Pharmacological profiles of selected atypical hallucinogens

	3,4-Methylenedioxy-methamphetamine (MDMA)	Salvinorin A	2C-I-NBOMe	2C-E	2C-T-7	3C-Bromo-dragonfly
Mechanism of action	Presynaptic release of 5-HT, dopamine, and norepinephrine; 5-HT reuptake inhibition	κ-Opioid agonism	5-HT_2 agonism/antagonism	5-HT_2 agonism/antagonism	5-HT_2 agonism/antagonism	5-HT_2 agonism/antagonism
Psychoactive dosing range	40–200 mg	250–750 mg (dried leaf)	50–1,500 μg	2–40 mg (oral); 1–10 mg (insufflated)	3–60 mg (oral); 1–25 mg (insufflated)	100–800 μg
Typical route(s) of ingestion	Oral; insufflation	Smoked	Sublingual; insufflation	Oral; insufflation	Oral; insufflation	Oral

TABLE 9–4. Pharmacological profiles of selected atypical hallucinogens *(continued)*

	3,4-Methylenedioxy-methamphetamine (MDMA)	Salvinorin A	2C-I-NBOMe	2C-E	2C-T-7	3C-Bromo-dragonfly
Time to onset	20–90 min	20–60 s	15–120 min	20–90 min (oral); 1–10 min (insufflated)	60–90 min (oral); 5–15 min (insufflated)	20–90 min
Approximate time to peak effect	2 h	2 min	1–2 h	2 h (oral); 30–60 min (insufflated)	2 h (oral); 30–60 min (insufflated)	2 h
Duration of effect	3–5 h	30–60 min	6–10 h	4–9 h (oral); 3–6 h (insufflated)	5–10 h (oral); 3–7 h (insufflated)	12–24 h

Note. 2C-E=2,5-dimethoxy-4-ethylphenethylamine; 2C-I-NBOMe=2-(4-iodo-2,5-dimethoxyphenyl)-N-[(2-methoxyphenyl)methyl]ethanamine; 2C-T-7=2,5-dimethoxy-4-*n*-propylthiophenethylamine; 3C-bromo-dragonfly=1-(8-bromobenzo[1,2-b;4,5-b']difuran-4-yl)-2-aminopropane; 5-HT=serotonin.

TABLE 9–5. Pharmacological profiles of selected dissociative drugs

	Phencyclidine (PCP)	Ketamine	Dextromethorphan (DXM)
Mechanism of action	NMDA antagonism	NMDA antagonism	NMDA antagonism
Psychoactive dosing range (mg)	3–10	10–250	100–1,500
Typical route(s) of ingestion	Smoked; insufflation; oral	Insufflation; intramuscular injection	Oral
Time to onset (min)	2–20	5–15	15–30
Approximate time to peak effect	1–2 h	30 min	90 min
Duration of effect	4–6 h	45–60 min	4–8 h (immediate release); 6–12 h (extended release)

Note. NMDA=*N*-methyl-D-aspartate.

Other substances that can yield false-positive PCP urine test results include

- Diphenhydramine
- Tramadol
- Meperidine
- Chlorpromazine
- Venlafaxine
- Lamotrigine
- Alprazolam
- Clonazepam
- Carvedilol

How to Recognize Intoxication

The typical user of a hallucinogen or dissociative drug presenting to a hospital setting is likely to be a white male younger than 30. The exception to this rule is PCP, for which approximately twice as many emergency department visits involve African American individuals (Table 9–2). That said, any presentation of severe anxiety, psychosis, disorganized behavior, or agitation in an otherwise healthy young person should raise suspicions for acute hallucinogen or dissociative drug intoxication, irrespective of gender or ethnicity. Sensorium is generally intact; most users have insight into the drug-induced nature of their experience and can report what they have ingested.

DSM-5 divides its "Hallucinogen-Related Disorders" section between PCP (and related substances such as ketamine and DXM; Box 9–1) and all "other" hallucinogens (Box 9–2). This is a helpful way of organizing one's clinical approach to a potentially intoxicated patient, because the toxidromes are considerably distinct.

Box 9–1. Diagnostic Criteria for Phencyclidine Intoxication

A. Recent use of phencyclidine (or a pharmacologically similar substance).
B. Clinically significant problematic behavioral changes (e.g., belligerence, assaultiveness, impulsiveness, unpredictability, psychomotor agitation, impaired judgment) that developed during, or shortly after, phencyclidine use.

C. Within 1 hour, two (or more) of the following signs or symptoms:

Note: When the drug is smoked, "snorted," or used intravenously, the onset may be particularly rapid.

1. Vertical or horizontal nystagmus.
2. Hypertension or tachycardia.
3. Numbness or diminished responsiveness to pain.
4. Ataxia.
5. Dysarthria.
6. Muscle rigidity.
7. Seizures or coma.
8. Hyperacusis.

D. The signs or symptoms are not attributable to another medical condition and are not better explained by another mental disorder, including intoxication with another substance.

Box 9–2.   Diagnostic Criteria for Other Hallucinogen Intoxication

A. Recent use of a hallucinogen (other than phencyclidine).
B. Clinically significant problematic behavioral or psychological changes (e.g., marked anxiety or depression, ideas of reference, fear of "losing one's mind," paranoid ideation, impaired judgment) that developed during, or shortly after, hallucinogen use.
C. Perceptual changes occurring in a state of full wakefulness and alertness (e.g., subjective intensification of perceptions, depersonalization, derealization, illusions, hallucinations, synesthesias) that developed during, or shortly after, hallucinogen use.
D. Two (or more) of the following signs developing during, or shortly after, hallucinogen use:

1. Pupillary dilation.
2. Tachycardia.
3. Sweating.
4. Palpitations.
5. Blurring of vision.
6. Tremors.
7. Incoordination.

E. The signs or symptoms are not attributable to another medical condition and are not better explained by another mental disorder, including intoxication with another substance.

As these criteria reflect, the hallucinogens and dissociative drugs all have a stimulatory effect on the sympathetic nervous system. For the classic hallucinogens, DXM, and ketamine, these effects are typically mild; the presence of severe vital sign abnormalities suggests intoxication with PCP, MDMA, a substituted phenethylamine, or a different class of substances altogether (e.g., cocaine or methamphetamine). Another consideration is serotonin syndrome, because all of the substances in this chapter, with the exception of PCP, ketamine, and *Salvia,* have enough serotonergic activity to precipitate serotonin syndrome when combined with other serotonergic agents.

The following subsections describe certain hallmark signs of intoxication specific to selected substances, which go beyond the generic features detailed in DSM-5.

MDMA INTOXICATION

- Hyperpyrexia (body temperature >40°C/104°F)
- Hyponatremia (secondary to both syndrome of inappropriate antidiuretic hormone secretion and increased water consumption)
- Bruxism/trismus (teeth grinding/jaw clenching)
- Cardiac arrhythmia
- Liver inflammation

Note that tablets sold on the street as "Ecstasy" are frequently adulterated with other substances, typically psychostimulants or dissociative drugs such as ketamine, PCP, amphetamine/methamphetamine, and caffeine.

DESIGNER DRUGS OR SUBSTITUTED PHENETHYLAMINE INTOXICATION

Because hundreds of designer drugs or substituted phenethylamines are currently in circulation, an exhaustive list of these and their effects is impractical. For specific information about a particular substance in this class, the reader is encouraged to visit the Web site www.erowid.org, which maintains an extensive and well-informed database for these compounds (and all the others in this chapter).

PHENCYCLIDINE INTOXICATION

- Constricted pupils—unique among hallucinogens and dissociative drugs
- Horizontal, vertical, or rotatory nystagmus

- "Acute brain syndrome"
  - Disorientation
  - Confusion
  - Inappropriate affect
  - Memory loss
- Frank psychosis
  - Auditory or visual hallucinations
  - Grandiose or paranoid delusions
  - Can be indistinguishable from acute schizophrenia; urine drug screen is key
- Agitation or violence
- Perseverative, purposeless, and bizarre behavior
- Catatonic stupor

PCP is highly lipid soluble and stored in fatty tissues on ingestion; subsequent mobilization from these stores results in a waxing and waning state of intoxication that can last for days or even weeks in heavy users.

KETAMINE INTOXICATION

- Moderately dilated pupils
- Horizontal, vertical, or rotatory nystagmus (less common than with PCP)
- Hypersalivation
- Petit mal seizures
- "K-Hole" (high doses)—an intense mind-body dissociation/out-of-body experience

DEXTROMETHORPHAN INTOXICATION

- Dilated pupils
- "Flanging"—a strobelike visual distortion, wherein moving objects take on a staccato appearance similar to stop-motion animation
- "Robo-walk"—a plodding, "zombielike" gait ataxia

What to Do About Intoxication

Except in cases of severe agitation or extreme medical complications, the management of acute hallucinogen or dissociative drug intoxication is largely supportive. The cornerstone of treatment is the removal of the patient to a calm, quiet, and subdued environment with a minimum of sensory stimulation, ideally in the presence of an empathetic and nonjudgmental staff member for periodic verbal reassurance until the self-limited effects of the intoxication run their course.

For severe agitation, pharmacological intervention with intravenous or intramuscular benzodiazepines is generally effective and well tolerated. Suggested agents and dosing parameters for agitation induced by intoxication with hallucinogens, as well as ketamine and DXM, are as follows (note that recommended doses for PCP intoxication are higher and are described later in their own section):

- Midazolam: 1–2 mg intravenously or intramuscularly
- Lorazepam: 1–2 mg intravenously or intramuscularly
- Diazepam: 2–5 mg intravenously or intramuscularly

Doses should be repeated every 3–5 minutes as needed until the patient is calm. Intravenous administration is preferable to intramuscular, so peripheral venous access should be established as soon as can be safely accomplished.

As a rule, antipsychotics (e.g., haloperidol 2–5 mg intravenously or intramuscularly; chlorpromazine 25 mg intravenously or intramuscularly) should be reserved only for severe agitation that is unresponsive to benzodiazepines because of their propensity to lower the seizure threshold and exacerbate complications such as hyperthermia. For these reasons, antipsychotics should be avoided altogether in cases of MDMA, ketamine, or DXM intoxication.

Beyond these general guidelines, additional special considerations for MDMA and the dissociative drugs are discussed in further detail below.

MDMA

1. Administer activated charcoal for severe intoxication if within 1 hour of ingestion.
2. Monitor vital signs for a minimum of 12 hours.

   - Treat symptomatic narrow complex tachycardia with β-blockers (only if cocaine intoxication has been ruled out), such as metoprolol 5–10 mg intravenously.
   - Treat hypertension with calcium channel blockers, such as nifedipine 5–10 mg by mouth, or α-adrenergic antag-

onists (only if cocaine intoxication has been ruled out), such as phentolamine 2–5 mg intravenously.

- In cases of hyperthermia/hyperpyrexia:

  - Patients may be hypotensive as a result of sweating-related volume losses; the priority here is to restore blood volume with intravenous normal saline.
  - At rectal temperatures greater than 106°F (41°C), sedation and active cooling (e.g., ice bath) should be pursued.
  - Beware of rhabdomyolysis and disseminated intravascular coagulation (DIC), for which risk increases with body temperature.

3. Use laboratory testing.

   - Serum sodium level

     - Symptomatic hyponatremia occurs at levels lower than 130 mmol/L—mental status changes are common.
     - Fluid restriction and supportive care typically suffice for minor cases.
     - Intravenous hypertonic saline is indicated in cases that are severe (serum sodium <125 mmol/L) or seriously symptomatic (e.g., seizures).

   - Liver function tests—rare cases of MDMA-related hepatitis have been reported, with severity of liver damage ranging from mild to massive.
   - Creatinine phosphokinase and urine myoglobin—to monitor for rhabdomyolysis
   - Platelet count, coagulation panel, and fibrin degradation products—to monitor for DIC

4. Beware of serotonin syndrome, which may be caused by MDMA alone or in combination with other serotonergic agents, characterized by the following:

   - Confusion or agitation
   - Hyperthermia or diaphoresis
   - Autonomic instability
   - Diarrhea
   - Increased muscle tone and deep tendon reflexes
   - Resolution typically occurs within 24 hours with sedation and supportive treatment. Severe cases can precipitate

- Seizure—treat with intravenous benzodiazepines
- Extreme hyperthermia—may require active cooling (e.g., ice bath) or paralysis and ventilation
- Must administer cyproheptadine for serotonin receptor blockade in either case

PHENCYCLIDINE

1. Make rapid control of severe psychomotor agitation a priority.
   - Physical restraints may be necessary.
   - Pharmacological sedation should be used as soon as possible.
     - Lorazepam 4 mg intravenously or intramuscularly
     - Diazepam 5–10 mg intravenously or intramuscularly
     - Midazolam 5 mg intravenously or intramuscularly
     - Repeat every 8–10 minutes until sedation is achieved.
2. Treat mild to moderate agitation with lower doses of benzodiazepines.
3. Carefully assess for trauma in patients with bizarre behavior and diminished pain perception.
4. Monitor vital signs for a minimum of 6 hours.
   - Hyperthermia typically resolves with adequate sedation.
   - Hypertension is typically transient and responds adequately to sedation—use short-acting agents (e.g., nitroglycerin or nitroprusside) for refractory cases.
5. Use laboratory testing.
   - Creatinine phosphokinase and urine myoglobin—to assess for rhabdomyolysis
   - Blood glucose—hypoglycemia is common
   - Liver function tests—transaminase elevation is common

KETAMINE

1. Monitor vital signs for 3–6 hours.
   - Cardiovascular effects rarely require intervention.
   - Extremely high doses may cause bradycardia.

- Treat with atropine 0.01–0.02 mg/kg intravenously (minimum dose=0.1 mg), repeated every 5 minutes as necessary, until a maximum total dose is 3 mg.
- Extreme hypersalivation may cause aspiration and respiratory compromise.
    - Treat with glycopyrrolate 5 µg/kg intravenously, repeated every 2–3 minutes as necessary, with maximum single and total doses of 0.2 mg and 0.8 mg, respectively.

2. Avoid laboratory testing—generally not useful in the absence of complicating clinical conditions.

DEXTROMETHORPHAN

1. Administer activated charcoal for severe intoxication if within 1 hour of ingestion.
2. Monitor vital signs for a minimum of 4–6 hours.
   - Cardiovascular effects rarely require intervention.
   - Hyperthermia typically resolves with adequate sedation.
3. Note that over-the-counter formulations of DXM frequently contain other agents that can complicate management in overdose, most importantly the following:
   - Acetaminophen—can precipitate liver failure
   - Antihistamines—can precipitate anticholinergic delirium
   - α_1-Adrenergic agonists (e.g., phenylephrine)—can precipitate hypertensive crisis
4. Be aware that respiratory depression and coma can occur at high doses, especially in a setting of co-ingestion with alcohol.
   - May be reversible with naloxone—0.1 mg/kg intravenously; maximum initial dose 2 mg
5. Use laboratory testing.
   - Blood alcohol level
   - Serum acetaminophen level
   - Liver function tests
6. Beware of serotonin syndrome, which may be caused by DXM alone or in combination with other serotonergic agents.

- See earlier section "MDMA" for clinical features and treatment recommendations.

How to Recognize Withdrawal

With the exception of MDMA, no established withdrawal syndromes are associated with any of the hallucinogens or dissociative drugs. MDMA use has been associated with a withdrawal syndrome consisting of mild dysphoria, anxiety, and insomnia lasting several days, but these symptoms are rarely severe enough to warrant clinical attention.

How to Recognize Addiction

As mentioned earlier, the classic hallucinogens, as well as *Salvia*, have virtually no addictive liability, although they can certainly be used in a manner that qualifies as abuse. The same is likely true for most of the substituted phenethyl-amines, although this is a tentative statement given the paucity of long-term epidemiological data regarding their use.

In contrast, abuse of dissociative drugs and, to a lesser extent, MDMA can induce craving and progress to a full-blown dependence syndrome, as described by the DSM-5 criteria in Boxes 9–3 and 9–4.

Box 9–3.   Diagnostic Criteria for Phencyclidine Use Disorder

---

A. A pattern of phencyclidine (or a pharmacologically similar sub-stance) use leading to clinically significant impairment or distress, as manifested by at least two of the following, occurring within a 12-month period:

  1. Phencyclidine is often taken in larger amounts or over a longer period than was intended.
  2. There is a persistent desire or unsuccessful efforts to cut down or control phencyclidine use.
  3. A great deal of time is spent in activities necessary to obtain phencyclidine, use the phencyclidine, or recover from its effects.
  4. Craving, or a strong desire or urge to use phencyclidine.
  5. Recurrent phencyclidine use resulting in a failure to fulfill major role obligations at work, school, or home (e.g., repeated

absences from work or poor work performance related to phencyclidine use; phencyclidine-related absences, suspensions, or expulsions from school; neglect of children or household).

6. Continued phencyclidine use despite having persistent or recurrent social or interpersonal problems caused or exacerbated by the effects of the phencyclidine (e.g., arguments with a spouse about consequences of intoxication; physical fights).

7. Important social, occupational, or recreational activities are given up or reduced because of phencyclidine use.

8. Recurrent phencyclidine use in situations in which it is physically hazardous (e.g., driving an automobile or operating a machine when impaired by a phencyclidine).

9. Phencyclidine use is continued despite knowledge of having a persistent or recurrent physical or psychological problem that is likely to have been caused or exacerbated by the phencyclidine.

10. Tolerance, as defined by either of the following:

    a. A need for markedly increased amounts of the phencyclidine to achieve intoxication or desired effect.

    b. A markedly diminished effect with continued use of the same amount of the phencyclidine.

Note: Withdrawal symptoms and signs are not established for phencyclidines, and so this criterion does not apply. (Withdrawal from phencyclidines has been reported in animals but not documented in human users.)

Specify if:

In early remission
In sustained remission

Specify if:

In a controlled environment

Specify current severity:

Mild: Presence of 2–3 symptoms.
Moderate: Presence of 4–5 symptoms.
Severe: Presence of 6 or more symptoms.

Box 9–4.   Diagnostic Criteria for Other Hallucinogen Use Disorder

---

A. A problematic pattern of hallucinogen (other than phencyclidine) use leading to clinically significant impairment or distress, as manifested by at least two of the following, occurring within a 12-month period:

1. The hallucinogen is often taken in larger amounts or over a longer period than was intended.
2. There is a persistent desire or unsuccessful efforts to cut down or control hallucinogen use.
3. A great deal of time is spent in activities necessary to obtain the hallucinogen, use the hallucinogen, or recover from its effects.
4. Craving, or a strong desire or urge to use the hallucinogen.
5. Recurrent hallucinogen use resulting in a failure to fulfill major role obligations at work, school, or home (e.g., repeated absences from work or poor work performance related to hallucinogen use; hallucinogen-related absences, suspensions, or expulsions from school; neglect of children or household).
6. Continued hallucinogen use despite having persistent or recurrent social or interpersonal problems caused or exacerbated by the effects of the hallucinogen (e.g., arguments with a spouse about consequences of intoxication; physical fights).
7. Important social, occupational, or recreational activities are given up or reduced because of hallucinogen use.
8. Recurrent hallucinogen use in situations in which it is physically hazardous (e.g., driving an automobile or operating a machine when impaired by the hallucinogen).
9. Hallucinogen use is continued despite knowledge of having a persistent or recurrent physical or psychological problem that is likely to have been caused or exacerbated by the hallucinogen.
10. Tolerance, as defined by either of the following:
    a. A need for markedly increased amounts of the hallucinogen to achieve intoxication or desired effect.
    b. A markedly diminished effect with continued use of the same amount of the hallucinogen.

Note: Withdrawal symptoms and signs are not established for hallucinogens, and so this criterion does not apply.

Specify **the particular hallucinogen.**

Specify if:

In early remission
In sustained remission

Specify if:

In a controlled environment

Specify current severity:

Mild: Presence of 2–3 symptoms.
Moderate: Presence of 4–5 symptoms.
Severe: Presence of 6 or more symptoms.

What to Do About Addiction

No pharmacotherapy can reduce cravings or otherwise specifically target addiction to dissociative drugs or MDMA, so
behavioral interventions are the mainstay of treatment. Patients should be referred to an addiction specialist for individual therapy, as well as to self-help groups such as Narcotics
Anonymous. Intensive outpatient or inpatient rehabilitation
programs should be considered in cases of frequent relapse.

Special Issues With
Psychiatric Comorbidities

Patients with a predisposition to psychotic illness, such as
those with a personal diagnosis or strong family history of bipolar disorder or schizophrenia, are particularly susceptible to
the adverse psychological effects of the hallucinogens and dissociative drugs. Because the age at which these substances are
most frequently abused—late adolescence and early adulthood—coincides with that at which an endogenous psychotic
illness typically begins to manifest, an episode of intoxication
can essentially precipitate a first-break psychosis in a patient
with this vulnerability and thus a diagnosis of psychotic illness
should be considered if psychotic symptoms persist after the
acute intoxication has resolved. In such cases, admission to an
inpatient psychiatric unit for stabilization and treatment is the
standard of care.

Hallucinogen Persisting Perception Disorder

In a small minority of hallucinogen users, intermittent visual
disturbances after use can occur for days to weeks or even
years. When these symptoms cause significant distress or impairment, they are defined in DSM-5 as hallucinogen persisting perception disorder (Box 9–5).

Box 9–5. Diagnostic Criteria for Hallucinogen Persisting Perception Disorder

A. Following cessation of use of a hallucinogen, the reexperiencing of one or more of the perceptual symptoms that were experienced while intoxicated with the hallucinogen (e.g., geometric hallucinations, false perceptions of movement in the peripheral visual fields, flashes of color, intensified colors, trails of images of moving objects, positive afterimages, halos around objects, macropsia and micropsia).

B. The symptoms in Criterion A cause clinically significant distress or impairment in social, occupational, or other important areas of functioning.

C. The symptoms are not attributable to another medical condition (e.g., anatomical lesions and infections of the brain, visual epilepsies) and are not better explained by another mental disorder (e.g., delirium, major neurocognitive disorder, schizophrenia) or hypnopompic hallucinations.

This disorder is associated most frequently with LSD use and can occur after a single exposure. Common triggers include cannabis use and low light conditions. When reassurance that the condition is benign and will resolve spontaneously over time proves insufficient to allay a patient's anxiety, benzodiazepines can be used—and confer the added benefit of improving the condition itself in some cases.

KEY POINTS

The classic hallucinogens are a unique class of substances that are not addictive or lethal in overdose, but if used irresponsibly, can have devastating psychological consequences. Other types of hallucinogens and dissociative drugs are lethal in overdose and have addictive potential.

Hallucinogens and dissociative drugs account for a small fraction of acute presentations for substance intoxication. Among these, phencyclidine and 3,4-methylenedioxymethamphetamine (MDMA) are the most likely to require emergent medical attention and confer the highest risk for dangerous medical complications.

In the absence of serious complications, treatment of hallucinogen and dissociative drug intoxication is largely supportive. Benzodiazepines are the treatment of choice for severe agitation.

No clinically significant withdrawal syndromes are associated with any of the hallucinogens and dissociative drugs, although MDMA and dissociative drugs do possess addictive liability. Behavioral interventions are the only existing mode of treatment.

References

American Psychiatric Association: Diagnostic and Statistical Manual of Mental Disorders, 5th Edition. Arlington, VA, American Psychiatric Association, 2013

Holland J (ed): Ecstasy: The Complete Guide: A Comprehensive Look at the Risks and Benefits of MDMA. Rochester, VT, Park Street Press, 2001

Johnston LD, O'Malley PM, Miech RA, et al: Monitoring the Future national survey results on drug use: 1975–2014: Overview, key findings on adolescent drug use. Ann Arbor, Institute for Social Research, The University of Michigan, 2015. Available at: http://www.monitoringthefuture.org/pubs/monographs/mtf-overview2014.pdf. Accessed February 26, 2016.

National Institute on Drug Abuse: NIDA Research Report Series: Hallucinogens and Dissociative Drugs (NIH Publication No. 15-4209). Revised February 2015. Available at: https://d14rmgtrwzf5a.cloudfront.net/sites/default/files/hallucinogensrrs4.pdf. Accessed February 25, 2016.

Nichols DE: Hallucinogens. Pharmacol Ther 101(2):131–181, 2004 14761703

CHAPTER 10

Inhalants

ABIGAIL J. HERRON, D.O.

INHALANTS are a chemically diverse group of breathable chemicals that can be self-administered as gases or vapors. Some members of the class have medical indications, and are under the regulation of the U.S. Food and Drug Administration, but these and others are also abused as intoxicants, whereby they are deliberately inhaled to cause a high. Inhalants include many different types of compounds, several of which are widely available and easily purchased, such as gasoline and household cleaners (see Table 10–1).

Inhalants are known by many names, including

- Whippets
- Poppers
- Huff
- Bang
- Kick
- Sniff

More than 22 million Americans age 12 or older have used inhalants. Inhalant use is most prevalent among 12- to 17-year-olds, with inhalants being the fourth most common substance of abuse in this population, behind only alcohol, tobacco, and marijuana. Approximately 10% of adolescents have abused inhalants at some point. The pattern of inhalant use differs from that of most other substances, with use actually decreasing from eighth to twelfth grade. Although many individuals do not continue use from adolescence into adulthood, about half of the current users report duration of use of more than 1–2 years. The prevalence of inhalant use in adulthood falls considerably behind more commonly abused substances such as marijuana, cocaine, and opiates but still represents a

TABLE 10–1. Sources of inhalants

Product	Possible contents
Air freshener	Amyl, butyl, cyclohexyl nitrite; butane
Lighter fluid	Butane
Household cleaners	*n*-Hexane, tetrachloroethylene, xylene
Gasoline	Benzene, toluene, xylene (lead)
Hair spray	Butane, propane
Nail polish remover	Acetone, toluene
Paint thinner	Toluene, trichloroethylene, xylene
Markers	Xylene
Refrigerant	Freon
Rubber cement	Acetone, benzene, *n*-hexane, toluene
Spray paint	Butane, propane, toluene
Whipped cream canisters	Nitrous oxide

significant minority of adult substance abusers. Additionally, experimentation with inhalants during adolescence has been shown to be a risk factor for continued use of illicit drugs later in life. Abuse of inhalants is even more common outside the United States, particularly in developing countries among children who are disenfranchised.

The abuse liability of inhalants among adolescents is related to the following factors:

- Quick acting
- Short duration
- Free or low cost
- Easily available
- Generally not prosecuted
- Difficult to test for
- Not perceived as dangerous

Pharmacology

The abused inhalants include compounds that individuals self-administer as gases, vapors, and aerosols. Shared features of inhalants include the following:

- Highly lipophilic
- Rapidly absorbed through the lungs
- Cross the blood-brain barrier
- Accumulate in the brain, liver, and fatty tissue
- Some undergo hepatic metabolism, whereas others are excreted largely unchanged
- Onset of action is rapid, and duration is short
- Effects are potentiated by alcohol and benzodiazepines

Inhalants differ from most other classes of abusable substances in that they are grouped by their method of administration rather than shared effects. Inhalants are divided into three groups based on shared pharmacological properties:

1. Volatile alkyl nitrites
2. Nitrous oxide
3. Volatile solvents, fuels, and anesthetics

VOLATILE ALKYL NITRITES

The prototype of the volatile alkyl nitrites is amyl nitrite, which is used medically as a vasodilator in the treatment of angina. Amyl nitrite was once available over the counter and is supplied in liquid ampules that are broken open with a popping sound, giving them the street name "poppers" (Balster 2014). These compounds do not produce acute intoxication like that seen with the volatile solvents (see "Volatile Solvents, Fuels, and Anesthetics" later in this section). They are likely abused because of 1) their ability to produce syncope and 2) their effects on smooth muscles and tumescence, leading to their reputation as sexual enhancers.

NITROUS OXIDE

Nitrous oxide, also known as "laughing gas," is a commonly used gaseous anesthetic and is also available in whipped cream propellants sold for household use. The canisters, such as those used for filling balloons, can be diverted for abuse.

When the inhalant is taken in this way, users breathe almost 100% nitrous oxide, which can lead to anoxia. It has been shown to have reinforcing effects in both humans and animals, acting on multiple neurotransmitter systems, including opioids and γ-aminobutyric acid, and produces euphoria and feelings of intoxication.

VOLATILE SOLVENTS, FUELS, AND ANESTHETICS

Volatile solvents, fuels, and anesthetics are a chemically diverse group of inhalants, found in compounds such as paint thinner, polish removers, dry-cleaning fluids, and glues. They can produce a rapid-onset, short-lived, alcohol-like intoxication. Ethanol is also a solvent and can produce an anesthesia-like state at very high blood levels, although it is much less potent than other solvents for acute central nervous system effects. Volatile solvents and alcohol share pharmacological and behavioral effects with other depressant drugs such as sedatives.

ROUTES OF ADMINISTRATION

Inhalation is typically achieved through "sniffing," "bagging," or "huffing." *Sniffing* involves the inhalation of vapors directly from an open container. *Bagging* is inhalation of vapors from a plastic or paper bag, and *huffing* involves the inhalation of vapors by holding a piece of fabric that has been soaked in the volatile substance against the nose and mouth.

How to Recognize Intoxication

Although most of the substances in this class produce depressant-like effects, a much wider array of symptoms has been reported, including hallucinations, tremors, and seizures. Users experience a diverse set of effects depending on the substance used. Intoxication with inhalants is of shorter duration than with other drugs of abuse because of rapid absorption and elimination, although prolonged use can result in accumulation in muscle, skin, and fat, leading to a longer duration of intoxication. Symptoms of inhalant intoxication include

- Euphoria
- Disinhibition

- Dizziness/light-headedness
- Slurred speech
- Ataxia
- Drowsiness
- Increased incidence of accidents and injuries

The prototypical patient is an adolescent male who presents with odor of paint or solvents, a "glue sniffer's rash" around nose and mouth, conjunctival irritation and cough, nasal discharge, dyspnea, rales, or rhonchi.

At high levels of use, or when inhalants are used in combination with alcohol or other sedatives, toxic effects and overdose can be seen. Symptoms include

- Shortness of breath
- Dizziness or fainting
- Respiratory depression
- Arrhythmias
- Chest pain
- Vague muscle and joint pain
- Asphyxia, cardiac arrest, and death

When a user loses consciousness but continues to be exposed to the inhalant, lethal concentrations can accumulate in the brain. The cause of most overdose deaths is respiratory depression or suffocation.

Acute cardiotoxicity, also known as "sudden sniffing death," can result from increased sensitivity of the myocardium to catecholamines, which can occur when an intoxicated individual engages in strenuous activity.

Box 10–1 contains DSM-5 criteria for inhalant intoxication (American Psychiatric Association 2013).

Box 10–1.   Diagnostic Criteria for Inhalant Intoxication

A. Recent intended or unintended short-term, high-dose exposure to inhalant substances, including volatile hydrocarbons such as toluene or gasoline.

B. Clinically significant problematic behavioral or psychological changes (e.g., belligerence, assaultiveness, apathy, impaired judgment) that developed during, or shortly after, exposure to inhalants.

C. Two (or more) of the following signs or symptoms developing during, or shortly after, inhalant use or exposure:

1. Dizziness.
2. Nystagmus.
3. Incoordination.
4. Slurred speech.
5. Unsteady gait.
6. Lethargy.
7. Depressed reflexes.
8. Psychomotor retardation.
9. Tremor.
10. Generalized muscle weakness.
11. Blurred vision or diplopia.
12. Stupor or coma.
13. Euphoria.

D. The signs or symptoms are not attributable to another medical condition and are not better explained by another mental disorder, including intoxication with another substance.

What to Do About Intoxication

Because of the short duration and rapid recovery most commonly seen with inhalant use, little medical intervention is generally needed for acute intoxication. Unless comatose, users are rarely brought to the emergency department. When this does occur, however, treatment should include

- Securing the airway and ensuring adequate ventilation, including supplemental oxygen. In some cases, steroids can be helpful if severe bronchospasm is seen.
- Removing clothing or other items that may be saturated with solvent to prevent worsening of intoxication and protect medical personnel.
- Placing individuals on cardiac monitoring and treating for hypotension if present.
- Measuring electrolytes and replenishing as needed.

How to Recognize Withdrawal

Inhalant withdrawal is not recognized as a formal disorder in DSM-5. Reports of symptoms of withdrawal, however, include irritability, anxiety, poor attention and concentration, and craving, persisting up to several weeks after cessation of use. Other individuals have reported headaches, nausea or vomiting, hallucinations, runny eyes or nose, fast heartbeat, depressed mood, and anxiety during withdrawal from inhalants.

What to Do About Withdrawal

Treatment of withdrawal is supportive and focuses on symptomatic treatment with agents such as analgesics and antinausea medications or benzodiazepines for agitation or anxiety. Withdrawal symptoms tend to be self-limited. Research is very limited, and this area requires further study.

How to Recognize Addiction

Inhalants produce less physical dependence than other substances of abuse, and signs of addiction are largely behavioral. Tolerance does not appear to be a prominent feature of inhalant use. Regular users of inhalants clearly can develop a pattern of uncontrolled use, marked by a devotion of considerable time and effort to obtaining and using inhalants. Few tests are available for detection of inhalant use, and those tests that are available have narrow windows of detection, making clinical history essential to a diagnosis of inhalant use. Studies have shown a clear progression from early inhalant use to later use of drugs such as cocaine and heroin, and it is not uncommon for inhalant users to abuse other substances.

Some indicators of inhalant abuse include

- Paint or stains on the body or clothing
- Hidden rags, cloths, or empty containers
- Spots or sores around the mouth or nose
- Red or runny eyes and nose
- A chemical odor on the breath
- A dazed or dizzy appearance
- Loss of appetite
- Excitability
- Irritability
- Problems in school

- Memory loss
- General apathy

Box 10–2 contains DSM-5 criteria for inhalant use disorder.

Box 10–2. Diagnostic Criteria for Inhalant Use Disorder

A. A problematic pattern of use of a hydrocarbon-based inhalant substance leading to clinically significant impairment or distress, as manifested by at least two of the following, occurring within a 12-month period:

   1. The inhalant substance is often taken in larger amounts or over a longer period than was intended.
   2. There is a persistent desire or unsuccessful efforts to cut down or control use of the inhalant substance.
   3. A great deal of time is spent in activities necessary to obtain the inhalant substance, use it, or recover from its effects.
   4. Craving, or a strong desire or urge to use the inhalant substance.
   5. Recurrent use of the inhalant substance resulting in a failure to fulfill major role obligations at work, school, or home.
   6. Continued use of the inhalant substance despite having persistent or recurrent social or interpersonal problems caused or exacerbated by the effects of its use.
   7. Important social, occupational, or recreational activities are given up or reduced because of use of the inhalant substance.
   8. Recurrent use of the inhalant substance in situations in which it is physically hazardous.
   9. Use of the inhalant substance is continued despite knowledge of having a persistent or recurrent physical or psychological problem that is likely to have been caused or exacerbated by the substance.
   10. Tolerance, as defined by either of the following:
       a. A need for markedly increased amounts of the inhalant substance to achieve intoxication or desired effect.
       b. A markedly diminished effect with continued use of the same amount of the inhalant substance.

Specify **the particular inhalant:** When possible, the particular substance involved should be named (e.g., "solvent use disorder").

Specify if:
   In early remission
   In sustained remission
Specify if:
   In a controlled environment

Specify current severity:
   Mild: Presence of 2–3 symptoms.
   Moderate: Presence of 4–5 symptoms.
   Severe: Presence of 6 or more symptoms.

What to Do About Addiction

Evidence-based recommendations for the treatment of inhalant use disorder are lacking (Konghom et al. 2010). A combination of factors likely contributes to this, including lack of recognition among inhalant users about the extent of impairments, reluctance to seek treatment, lack of recognition by medical providers, and prevalence among adolescents, a population in which research trials are more burdensome.

When treating an inhalant use disorder, clinicians must rely on principles used in the treatment of other substance use disorders and apply those strategies. The following treatment principles should be used in the care of individuals with inhalant use disorder (National Inhalant Prevention Coalition 2015):

- The first step in treatment is a detailed history and physical examination. Given the heterogeneity of inhalants, and the difficulty in detecting these substances because of limitations in toxicology testing and short onset of action, history is particularly crucial in establishing an accurate picture of use, including which substances are used, and the frequency, duration, and method of use.

- Because many inhalants are stored in the fatty tissue of the body and are released over time, the inhalant user may continue to experience residual effects of use for days to even weeks after last use. These effects may extend the detoxification period beyond that which occurs with other substances of abuse.

- Substance use and psychiatric illness are often comorbid. Treatment of these co-occurring conditions should be a priority.

- Neurological impairment is often seen with chronic inhalant. These deficits may be primary or secondary to use and in either case can have a significant effect on an individual's ability to engage in treatment. Neurological testing can be helpful and should be repeated after several months of abstinence to help distinguish between acute and chronic impairments.

- Initial interventions should be very brief, informal, and concrete because the individual with inhalant use may have reduced attention span and impairment in complex thinking.
- Traditional talk or group therapy may not be appropriate for individuals with cognitive or behavioral impairments.

Special Issues With Psychiatric Comorbidities

High rates of psychiatric disorders have been reported among those abusing inhalants, with some studies reporting that 70% of inhalant users met criteria for at least one lifetime mood, anxiety, or personality disorder (Brouette and Anton 2001). Conduct disorder, mood disorders, and suicidality also are seen in adolescents with inhalant abuse, as well as increased rates of other substance use disorders. Evidence also suggests that these adolescents are more likely to have antisocial traits and a history of trauma compared with those who have never used inhalants (Ozden and Shah 2014).

Psychiatric effects of inhalant use include impaired judgment, confusion, fright, hyperactivity, anxiety, acute psychosis, increased violence and aggressive behavior, depression, organic brain syndrome, hallucinations, intellectual impairment, dementia, impulsivity, decreased attention, and withdrawal.

Treatment focuses on psychotherapy and pharmacotherapy for co-occurring psychiatric illness. As discussed earlier, individuals with inhalant use, particularly early in treatment or those with chronic neurological impairment, may have limitations in their ability to participate in talk or group therapy.

Special Issues With Medical Comorbidities

Inhalants, as a group, are potentially acutely toxic to multiple organ systems (as discussed earlier in the section "How to Recognize Intoxication") and can also cause widespread and long-lasting damage.

CHRONIC TOXICITY

Several factors make it difficult to determine the specific eti-ology of adverse effects seen in chronic inhalant users. Inhal-ants are a chemically diverse group composed of numerous substances, and many individuals engage in use of several different types of inhalants. Additionally, some commercially available products are composed of complex mixtures of chemicals, each of which has a distinct set of toxic effects. In-dividuals who engage in inhalant use can have other predic-tors of poor health outcomes, including homelessness, poor nutrition, co-occurring medical illness, and other substance use. Finally, much of the research into the effects of specific inhalant substances has focused on low-level, long-duration exposure that occurs in home or occupational use of chemi-cals rather than the repeated, intermittent, high-concentra-tion administration that occurs in inhalant misuse.

EFFECTS ON MAJOR ORGAN SYSTEMS

See Table 10–2 for a summary of effects of inhalants on major organ systems.

Chronic users of inhaled solvents can develop localized irritation of the eyes, nose, and mouth and experience skin rash, bleeding from the nose, rhinitis, and conjunctivitis. When these symptoms are accompanied by the odor of sol-vents on breath or clothing and/or staining from paint or sol-vents on face, hands, or clothing, these signs and symptoms are highly suggestive of inhalant misuse. Chronic inhalant use can lead to persistent cough, asthma-like symptoms, and impaired respiration.

Hepatic impairment also can be seen with chronic inhal-ant use because several inhaled chemicals are metabolized by the liver. Individuals with co-occurring substance use that can impair liver function or individuals with medical condi-tions affecting the liver, such as hepatitis, are especially vul-nerable.

NEUROTOXICITY

Many inhalants can cause significant damage to the nervous system, and the neurotoxic properties of some specific sub-stances have been well characterized. Although unleaded gasoline is now used in the United States, leaded gasoline is still used in many countries and produces classic demyelin-

TABLE 10–2. Adverse effects of inhalants on specific organ systems

Organ system	Adverse effects
Central nervous system	Encephalopathy
	Seizures
	Coma
	Cognitive dysfunction
	Dementia
	Decreased attention
	Impaired learning and information processing
	Apathy
	Poor memory
	Cerebellar damage
	Tremor
	Ataxia
	Peripheral neuropathy
	Trigeminal neuralgia
	Optic neuritis
	Delirium
	Impairment in working memory and executive functioning
Dermatological	Burns
	Perioral infection
	Rash
Cardiovascular	Arrhythmia
	Sudden sniffing death
	Cardiomyopathy
	Heart block

TABLE 10–2. Adverse effects of inhalants on specific organ systems *(continued)*

Organ system	Adverse effects
Renal	Renal tubular acidosis
	Urinary calculi
	Glomerulonephritis
	Hypokalemia
Pulmonary	Hypoxia
	Asphyxia
	Pneumonitis
	Emphysema
	Aspiration pneumonia
Hepatic	Hepatitis
	Hepatic failure
Hematopoietic	Bone marrow suppression
	Leukemia
	Lymphoma
	Aplastic anemia
	Multiple myeloma
Musculoskeletal	Rhabdomyolysis

ation. Imaging and autopsy of inhalant users show loss of white matter, brain atrophy, and damage to neural pathways. The prevalence of inhalant use during adolescence, a time during which the nervous system is still under development, is of particular concern.

Special Issues With Specific Populations

PREGNANCY

Inhalants cross the placenta, and use during pregnancy is associated with low birth weight, facial and other physical abnormalities, microcephaly, and delayed neurological and physical maturation. Because some features resemble those in fetal alcohol syndrome, a "fetal solvent syndrome" has been proposed. Decreased fertility and spontaneous abortions in some women also may be related to inhalant abuse.

ADOLESCENTS

As discussed earlier, inhalant use is particularly prevalent among adolescents, due in large part to the easy accessibility of these substances. Education about inhalants and the risks associated with use should be provided to children and adolescents. Supportive counseling, family therapy, and discussion in peer groups are important components of treatment.

KEY POINTS

Inhalant use is most prevalent among 12- to 17-year-olds, with inhalants being the fourth most common substance of abuse in this population, behind only alcohol, tobacco, and marijuana. Experimentation with inhalants during adolescence has been shown to be a risk factor for continued use of illicit drugs later in life.

Inhalants are a chemically diverse group of substances with differing effects, but common features of inhalants include rapid-onset, short-acting intoxication and an association between regular use and chronic neurological and other organ system impairment.

Because many inhalants are stored in the fatty tissue of the body and are released over time, the inhalant user may continue to experience residual effects of use for days to even weeks after last use.

Substance use and psychiatric illness are often comorbid. Treatment of these co-occurring conditions should be a priority. Neurological impairments that result from chronic inhalant use may make traditional talk therapy or group therapy difficult in this population.

References

American Psychiatric Association: Diagnostic and Statistical Manual of Mental Disorders, 5th Edition. Arlington, VA, American Psychiatric Association, 2013

Balster RL: Pharmacology of inhalants, in The ASAM Principles of Addiction Medicine, 5th Edition. Edited by Ries RK, Fiellin DA, Miller SC, et al. Philadelphia, PA, Lippincott Williams & Wilkins, 2014, pp 267–276

Brouette T, Anton R: Clinical review of inhalants. Am J Addict 10(1):79–94, 2001 11268830

Konghom S, Verachai V, Srisurapanont M, et al: Treatment for inhalant dependence and abuse. Cochrane Database Syst Rev 8(12):CD007537, 2010 21154379

National Inhalant Prevention Coalition Web site. Available at: http://www.inhalants.org. Accessed December 22, 2015.

Ozden A, Shah S: Inhalants, in The Addiction Casebook. Edited by Levounis P, Herron AJ. Washington, DC, American Psychiatric Publishing, 2014, pp 91–104

CHAPTER 11

Opioids

ERIN ZERBO, M.D.
RASHI AGGARWAL, M.D.

WIDELY used since ancient times, opioids are the oldest and most effective painkillers known. They induce euphoria and relieve both physical and emotional pain, resulting in reduced anxiety, anger, and sadness.

Synthesized by the pharmaceutical company Bayer in the late 1800s, heroin became illegal in the early 1900s once its addictive potential was realized. Around the same time, it became illegal for physicians to prescribe opioids to patients with known addiction.

It was not until the 1960s that methadone maintenance programs were created and allowed as an agonist treatment option for opioid use disorders. Buprenorphine also was approved for this use, in 2002, and methadone and buprenorphine remain the two opioid maintenance treatment options available today.

Today, a resurgence of heroin use is now being seen. Aggressive pharmaceutical marketing in the 1990s led to a marked increase in opioid prescribing for pain. Eventually charges of "criminal misbranding" and $600 million in fines resulted against Purdue Pharma, the makers of OxyContin, after it was found that they downplayed its risk of addiction (Van Zee 2009). Yet this verdict came too late: the opioid prescribing epidemic was already in full swing, and there has been a steady increase in opioid use and overdose deaths. Perhaps most concerning is a dramatic increase in opioid use among U.S. teenagers, with prescription opioids in the top of the list for "initiates" to illicit drug use in persons ages 12 and older (Substance Abuse and Mental Health Services Administration 2014). Individuals abusing or addicted to prescription opioids often switch to heroin because of its lower cost.

Public health interventions to target this opioid epidemic include marketing campaigns to increase awareness, more stringent regulations on opioid prescribing, and distribution of naloxone among law enforcement personnel to allow for a more timely response to overdose. "Take-home" naloxone kits are also distributed to opioid users themselves, with impressive data from Chicago, Illinois, showing decreased opioid overdose deaths citywide after the introduction of these kits. However, a serious deficit in availability of and access to opioid maintenance treatment persists, which is crucial to prevent overdose deaths and assist in long-term recovery for those who are already addicted. This is a major challenge in today's health care system.

Pharmacology

Opioids are derived from the opium poppy, *Papaver somniferum*. Raw opium is obtained by incising an opium seed pod and exposing its latex (juice), which dries on contact with air. The two commonly used terms are

1. *Opiates:* naturally occurring alkaloids found in the opium poppy (morphine, codeine, thebaine)
2. *Opioids:* both naturally occurring and synthetic opioids

Opioids bind to opioid receptors, found both centrally and peripherally (Ries et al. 2014). The three main opioid receptor subtypes are μ, κ, and δ (Table 11–1). Opioids can be categorized by origin or by function (Tables 11–2 and 11–3). In the brain, opioids inhibit γ-aminobutyric acid, leading to a burst of dopaminergic activity in the nucleus accumbens, which is the traditional "rush" associated with all abused drugs. Opioids have varying serum half-lives, ranging from several minutes (fentanyl-related opioids) to several hours (morphine) to several days (methadone, buprenorphine). For a list of commonly used opioids and their properties (including equianalgesic doses), see Table 11–4.

Opioids can be ingested by a variety of routes:

- Oral
- Intranasal ("sniffing")
- Intravenous injection ("shooting")

TABLE 11–1. Opioid receptor subtypes

Receptor subtype	Effect
μ	Most important for addiction and the clinical effects observed with opioids. Mediates addictive liability, euphoria, analgesia, miosis, respiratory depression, and reduced gastrointestinal motility.
κ	Dysphoria, analgesia, and psychedelic effects (note that the hallucinogen *Salvia divinorum* is a κ opioid agonist).
δ	Convulsant effects, mood effects, euphoria, and analgesia.

TABLE 11–2. Opioids classified by origin

Origin of opioid	Examples
Endogenous	Endorphins, enkephalins, endomorphins, dynorphins
Naturally occurring	Found in the opium poppy: morphine, codeine, thebaine
Semisynthetic	Requires synthesis from a naturally occurring opiate: heroin, buprenorphine, and many of the commonly prescribed opioid painkillers such as hydromorphone, hydrocodone, and oxycodone
Synthetic	Methadone, tramadol, fentanyl, meperidine

- Subcutaneous injection ("skin popping")
- Smoking, often on aluminum foil ("chasing the dragon")

TOXICOLOGY

Most routine urine immunoassays for opiates will detect morphine and related metabolites, including hydrocodone

TABLE 11–3. Opioids classified by function

Function of opioid	Examples
Pure agonist	Most marketed opioids, such as morphine, hydromorphone, oxycodone, fentanyl, methadone, and heroin (nearly all abused opioids are in this category)
Partial agonist	Buprenorphine, tramadol
Agonist-antagonist	Differing activity at opioid receptor subtypes; includes nalbuphine and pentazocine
Pure antagonist	Naloxone (liquid) and naltrexone (tablet), nalmefene

and hydromorphone; however, such testing is less sensitive for oxycodone (thus resulting in a false-negative result for this agent).

- Heroin is metabolized to 6-monoacetylmorphine (and morphine, so it would be detected on the standard opiates assay.
- Synthetic and some semisynthetic opioids (such as methadone and buprenorphine, respectively) require a specific immunoassay for detection.

Urine detection times generally range from 2 to 4 days, depending on the opioid. Because poppy seeds do contain naturally occurring opiates, their ingestion can indeed lead to a false-positive urine opiate screen result. Other types of toxicology screening are also available (serum, hair, oral fluid, sweat), although they are usually employed in forensic or workplace settings.

How to Recognize Intoxication

The classic "triad" of opioid overdose is

1. Decreased level of consciousness
2. Respiratory depression (<12 breaths/minute)
3. Miotic pupils

TABLE 11–4. Equianalgesic doses for commonly used opioids

Opioid	Dosing interval	Equianalgesic dose (mg, parenteral)	Equianalgesic dose (mg, oral)
Codeine	Every 3–4 h	130	200–300
Morphine	Every 3–4 h	10	30
Methadone	Every 6–8 h (or daily for maintenance)	10 (acute use)	20 (acute use)
Buprenorphine	Every 6–8 h (or daily for maintenance)	0.3	0.4 (sublingual)
Hydrocodone	Every 3–4 h	—	30
Hydromorphone	Every 3–4 h	1.5	7.5
Meperidine	Every 2–3 h	75	300
Oxycodone	Every 3–4 h	—	20

Other signs include

- Slurred speech
- Impaired attention and memory
- Behavioral changes (either psychomotor retardation or agitation)
- Scarred peripheral veins ("track marks") or skin infections in an intravenous user

Box 11–1 contains DSM-5 criteria for opioid intoxication (American Psychiatric Association 2013).

Box 11–1. Diagnostic Criteria for Opioid Intoxication

A. Recent use of an opioid.

B. Clinically significant problematic behavioral or psychological changes (e.g., initial euphoria followed by apathy, dysphoria, psychomotor agitation or retardation, impaired judgment) that developed during, or shortly after, opioid use.

C. Pupillary constriction (or pupillary dilation due to anoxia from severe overdose) and one (or more) of the following signs or symptoms developing during, or shortly after, opioid use:

1. Drowsiness or coma.
2. Slurred speech.
3. Impairment in attention or memory.

D. The signs or symptoms are not attributable to another medical condition and are not better explained by another mental disorder, including intoxication with another substance.

Specify if:

With perceptual disturbances

OBTAINING THE HISTORY

The clinician should determine opioid use (type of drug, amount, method of use, last use) and any other concurrent alcohol or drug use. He or she should collect collateral information from the patient's family, friends, or medical records. Given the changing demographics of opioid use, the clinician should not assume that a patient is not a user. A nonjudgmental attitude goes a long way in obtaining an accurate history.

TOLERANCE

Tolerance develops for cardiovascular and respiratory effects; hence patients are at greater risk for overdose on relapse after a period of abstinence and at lower risk for overdose with chronic use. Tolerance is less likely to develop for miosis or constipation. Chronic users can appear alert and oriented, with miosis being the only telltale sign of use.

What to Do About Intoxication

Respiratory depression is the primary concern. If the patient appears sedated with decreased ventilation, he or she should be monitored in a medical setting.

NALOXONE

Naloxone is an opioid antagonist that is used to reverse opioid overdose. Naloxone 0.4–0.8 mg is administered intranasally, subcutaneously, intramuscularly, or intravenously initially and repeated as necessary. If a significant withdrawal syndrome occurs, patients may become acutely combative and highly irritable. An aerosol spray form of naloxone is also available, which allows for a slower titration and is less likely to precipitate a severe withdrawal syndrome. The half-life of naloxone is 30–80 minutes, so it is important to observe for recurrence of intoxication or overdose once its effects wear off. All patients should be observed for 2–3 hours after naloxone is administered. Patients who have used longer-acting opioids such as methadone may need a naloxone infusion and continued monitoring (Nelson et al. 2010).

Take-home naloxone kits are now increasingly available to prescribe directly to opioid users. Such kits contain naloxone along with intramuscular needles or an intranasal apparatus, alcohol swabs, latex gloves, and instructions for use. They allow a layperson to administer naloxone at the time of an overdose in the community while 911 is being called. Given that naloxone is inactive in the absence of opioids, this is a safe intervention, and data show that it seems to be effective in reducing overdose deaths. Many local and state governments are now passing laws to allow the distribution of take-home naloxone kits to users (either with or without a doctor's prescription), with the goal that such users will go on to train their friends and family.

MEDICAL WORKUP

Clinicians should rule out hypoglycemia, fluid and electrolyte abnormalities, hepatic encephalopathy, HIV-related opportunistic infections, and any other potential etiologies for an altered mental status relevant to the patient's history and presentation. Prolonged hypoxia can result in rhabdomyolysis, myocardial infarction, and central nervous system (CNS) injury (Nelson et al. 2010).

Clinicians should obtain a toxicology screen and a blood alcohol level and consider concurrent intoxication with another substance. Benzodiazepine use is common among opioid-using individuals and may not be detectable on a urine toxicology screen; flumazenil can be used to reverse overdose. If illicit opioids are involved, the patient may have ingested adulterants, such as dextromethorphan, lidocaine, and scopolamine.

How to Recognize Withdrawal

Acute opioid withdrawal is the most subjectively uncomfortable of all the withdrawal syndromes, but it is not fatal under usual circumstances. In patients with severe cardiovascular or respiratory illness who cannot tolerate large fluid shifts, it does have the potential to be fatal.

Opioid withdrawal has two phases:

1. Acute withdrawal (hours to days)
2. Protracted abstinence syndrome (weeks to months, and perhaps even years)

Acute withdrawal is essentially the physiological "rebound" of organ systems that have been altered by the presence of opioids. Because opioids suppress CNS function in intoxication, their absence leads to CNS hyperactivity in withdrawal. One example is the significant noradrenergic hyperactivity that emerges from the locus coeruleus during opioid withdrawal, which can be suppressed by the noradrenergic agonist clonidine.

Clinicians should use the Clinical Opiate Withdrawal Scale (COWS; Wesson and Ling 2003) to assess for acute withdrawal symptoms; Table 11–5 shows the items rated and their scoring. COWS can be used to quantify the severity and guide the treatment of opioid withdrawal in someone known or suspected to have opioid dependence, much as the Clinical Institute Withdrawal Assessment is used for alcohol withdrawal. The first symptom is often anxiety, and anticipation of withdrawal symptoms can lead to actual physiological withdrawal itself.

Box 11–2 contains DSM-5 criteria for opioid withdrawal.

Box 11–2. Diagnostic Criteria for Opioid Withdrawal

A. Presence of either of the following:

1. Cessation of (or reduction in) opioid use that has been heavy and prolonged (i.e., several weeks or longer).
2. Administration of an opioid antagonist after a period of opioid use.

B. Three (or more) of the following developing within minutes to several days after Criterion A:

1. Dysphoric mood.
2. Nausea or vomiting.
3. Muscle aches.
4. Lacrimation or rhinorrhea.
5. Pupillary dilation, piloerection, or sweating.
6. Diarrhea.
7. Yawning.
8. Fever.
9. Insomnia.

C. The signs or symptoms in Criterion B cause clinically significant distress or impairment in social, occupational, or other important areas of functioning.

D. The signs or symptoms are not attributable to another medical condition and are not better explained by another mental disorder, including intoxication or withdrawal from another substance.

Other acute withdrawal symptoms not mentioned in COWS or DSM-5 criteria include:

- Anorexia
- Opioid craving
- Hypertension
- Abdominal pain
- Myoclonus (hence the phrase "kicking the habit")
- Sneezing

The severity of withdrawal depends on the type and dose of opioid, along with the duration of use. Injection use has been associated with more severe withdrawal. The timing of withdrawal symptoms is determined by the half-life of the

TABLE 11–5. Items rated in the Clinical Opiate Withdrawal Scale (COWS)

Resting pulse rate *(after patient is sitting/lying for 1 minute)*

(0) pulse rate 80 or below; (1) pulse rate 81–100;
(2) pulse rate 101–120; (4) pulse rate >120

Sweating *(over past 30 minutes, not accounted for by room temperature or patient activity)*

(0) no report of chills or flushing; (1) subjective report of chills or flushing; (2) flushed or observable moistness on face; (3) beads of sweat on brow or face; (4) sweat streaming off face

Restlessness *(observed during assessment)*

(0) able to sit still; (1) subjective report of difficulty sitting still, but is able to do so; (3) frequent shifting or extraneous movements of legs/arms; (5) unable to sit still for more than few seconds

Pupil size

(0) pupils pinned or normal size for room light; (1) slightly dilated pupils; (2) pupils moderately dilated; (5) pupils dilated such that only rim of iris visible

Bone or joint aches *(attributable to opioid withdrawal only)*

(0) not present; (1) mild diffuse discomfort; (2) subjective report of severe diffuse aching of joints/muscles;
(4) patient is rubbing joints/muscles and is unable to sit still because of discomfort

Running nose/lacrimation *(not accounted for by cold/ allergies)*

(0) not present; (1) nasal stuffiness or unusually moist eyes; (2) nose running or tearing; (4) nose running constantly and/or tears streaming down face

GI upset *over last 30 minutes*

(0) no GI symptoms; (1) stomach cramps; (2) nausea or loose stools; (3) any vomiting or diarrhea; (5) multiple episodes of vomiting or diarrhea

Tremor *(observe outstretched arms/hands)*

(0) no tremor; (1) tremor can be felt, but not observed;
(2) slight tremor observable; (4) gross tremor or muscle twitching

TABLE 11–5. Items rated in the Clinical Opiate Withdrawal Scale (COWS) *(continued)*

Yawning *(observe during assessment)*

(0) no yawning; (1) yawning 1–2 times during assessment; (2) yawning 3+ times during assessment; (4) yawning several times per minute

Anxiety or irritability

(0) none; (1) patient reports increasing irritability or anxiety; (2) patient obviously irritable or anxious; (4) patient so irritable or anxious that participation in assessment is difficult

Gooseflesh skin

(0) none/skin is smooth; (3) palpable piloerection or hairs felt standing up on arms; (5) prominent piloerection

Scoring

5–12=mild; 13–24=moderate; 25–36=moderately severe; 37+=severe withdrawal

Source. Adapted from Wesson and Ling 2003.

opioid: withdrawal can begin as early as 4–6 hours after the last use of heroin or as late as 36 hours after the last use of methadone.

- Heroin withdrawal peaks within 36–72 hours and can last up to 10 days.
- Methadone withdrawal peaks in 72–96 hours and can last up to 25 days.

A protracted abstinence syndrome has been supported by observations of physiological dysfunction that can take 6 months or more to return to baseline function. Persistent changes have been noted in blood pressure, heart rate, body temperature, and pupil size, along with decreased sensitivity to carbon dioxide, increased sedimentation rates, and electroencephalographic changes. It is hypothesized that this syndrome contributes significantly to the high relapse rate in opioid users, because it likely results in psychological discomfort and increased opioid cravings.

What to Do About Withdrawal

Withdrawal should be treated immediately. Allowing patients to experience withdrawal in order to provide negative reinforcement or punishment is not helpful or ethical. Timely treatment will help to establish a good rapport with the patient, and this increases the chance of connection to appropriate aftercare. Opioid-dependent patients often have had negative experiences with health care providers, so approaching these patients with respect and empathy can go a long way.

The two options to treat withdrawal are

1. Opioid replacement
2. Nonopioid treatment for symptomatic relief

OPIOID REPLACEMENT

Any opioid will provide relief from opioid withdrawal, but when we know a patient has an opioid use disorder, we choose either methadone or buprenorphine (as per patient and/or physician preference). A federal "3-day rule" (Title 21 CFR, Part 1306) established that opioids should not be administered for detoxification for more than 72 hours if the prescriber is not part of a narcotic treatment program. However, this rule was not meant to obstruct medical care, so an extended detoxification period is allowed if medically necessary. This is often the case during an inpatient medical/surgical admission; the detoxification period can be as short as 2–3 days, but can be prolonged if needed. Either methadone or buprenorphine can be used for detoxification. Although buprenorphine prescribing normally requires a special waiver, this is not required when the patient has an acute medical condition that would be complicated by withdrawal. The waiver is required for maintenance treatment.

Methadone maintenance requires enrollment in a licensed methadone clinic, so methadone maintenance cannot be initiated in the hospital; on the other hand, buprenorphine maintenance can be provided by any practitioner with a Drug Addiction Treatment Act (DATA) of 2000 waiver, and so it can be initiated during the hospital stay. Maintenance is always preferable to detoxification, because relapse rates approach 95%. For further information on maintenance treatment, see the section "What To Do About Addiction" later in this chapter.

METHADONE

Clinicians should start methadone with 10–20 mg orally for the first dose and give an additional 5–10 mg if withdrawal symptoms persist after 1 hour. No more than 30 mg should be given as the first dose, and 40 mg total should not be exceeded in the first day. Dosing can be once or twice per day. The dose can be reduced by 50% per day if the goal is a 3-day taper, or more slowly if a longer taper is preferred. Methadone has a long half-life and it takes 3–5 days to achieve a steady state level, so the serum level will continue to increase even if the patient receives the same dose each day.

A 30-mg dose of methadone will not cause respiratory depression even in a patient who is entirely naive to opioids. A 20-mg dose of methadone should treat the most severe withdrawal symptoms for every patient, even if the patient normally consumes a large quantity of opioids.

It is important to note that an individual physician *cannot* start a patient on methadone maintenance and then refer the patient to a methadone clinic. A patient must be accepted into a methadone clinic first and then methadone can be titrated and continued.

BUPRENORPHINE

Clinicians should start buprenorphine with a 2- to 4-mg dose when the patient has moderate withdrawal symptoms and titrate up to a maximum of 12–16 mg in the first day in divided 4-mg doses. It is important to alert the patient that buprenorphine is sublingual and will not be absorbed if it is swallowed. After the patient is stabilized on the appropriate dose for 2 days, buprenorphine should be tapered over 3–6 days (or longer if possible). The entire detoxification can be accomplished in 72 hours if necessary, simply by reducing the dose by 50% per day.

Clinicians should wait until the patient has *moderate* withdrawal symptoms before giving the first dose: 12–16 hours after short-acting opioids such as heroin or 48–96 hours after a long-acting opioid such as methadone (although this estimate is for patients who have been maintained on daily methadone; if a patient has been taking methadone inconsistently, a shorter time would suffice).

Buprenorphine is a partial agonist, so the receptors will be activated at a diminished level as compared with full agonists such as methadone, heroin, and most prescription opioids. Because buprenorphine has one of the highest affinities for the opioid receptor, it will displace these other full agonists and cause a precipitated withdrawal syndrome if given too early. If precipitated withdrawal does occur, clinicians should give additional buprenorphine and titrate more quickly and consider nonopioid adjuncts for withdrawal (see the next section, "Nonopioid Treatment"). Clinicians should not revert to treatment with another opioid, because of pharmacodynamic interactions with buprenorphine, which is already present. Withdrawal symptoms should improve with additional buprenorphine because a greater number of opioid receptors will become occupied.

If a patient is admitted to the hospital for a medical condition and experiences opioid withdrawal while in the hospital, the physician does *not* need a DATA 2000 waiver to use buprenorphine, because withdrawal may complicate the medical condition and is therefore considered urgent. An outpatient referral to a physician with a DATA waiver should be arranged for maintenance treatment with buprenorphine. See "What to Do About Addiction" for further details on the DATA 2000 waiver.

NONOPIOID TREATMENT

Nonopioid agents have been shown to be effective in treating opioid withdrawal.

CLONIDINE

Clinicians should start clonidine at 0.1 mg every 4–6 hours as needed for withdrawal symptoms. The dose can be increased by 0.1–0.2 mg/day to a maximum of 1.2 mg (the average maximum dose is 0.8 mg). Blood pressure should be monitored because side effects include hypotension and sedation. A typical course is 7–10 days, with a taper by 0.1–0.2 mg/day toward the end to avoid rebound hypertension and headaches. Clonidine can also be used for a 3-day taper if needed. Often, clonidine is used as needed during an opioid agonist taper, providing additional relief from any residual withdrawal symptoms (Ries et al. 2014).

Clonidine is a centrally acting α_2-adrenergic agonist that inhibits the increased norepinephrine outflow from the locus coeruleus that occurs during opioid withdrawal, therefore helping to alleviate autonomic signs and symptoms. It is less effective for subjective withdrawal symptoms and does not address anxiety, restlessness, insomnia, or muscle aches. Although significant literature on clonidine detoxification exists, patients seem to prefer detoxification with opioid agonists, and retention rates are generally higher in detoxification studies that use opioid agonists.

Yet clonidine does have advantages: it is not a controlled substance, it has a minimal risk of diversion, and physicians with less experience with methadone or buprenorphine will likely feel comfortable prescribing it. Other α_2-adrenergic agonists such as guanfacine also may be considered; lofexidine, an analogue of clonidine, is not approved for use in the United States but is used extensively for opioid withdrawal in the United Kingdom and seems to be just as effective as clonidine, with fewer side effects.

OTHER AGENTS

Tramadol (600 mg/day) was found to relieve objective opioid withdrawal symptoms. One study showed promise for memantine (20 mg/day). Higher doses of gabapentin (1,600 mg/day) also were found to be helpful (Ries et al. 2014).

ADJUNCTS FOR SYMPTOMATIC RELIEF

- Ibuprofen or other nonsteroidal anti-inflammatory drugs for myalgias
- Loperamide or other antimotility agents for diarrhea
- Ondansetron or other antiemetics for nausea and vomiting
- Diazepam, clonazepam, or other benzodiazepines for restlessness and insomnia

Anesthesia-assisted ultrarapid opioid detoxification, in which high doses of naloxone are administered under anesthesia, allows the patient to be detoxified without consciously experiencing withdrawal symptoms. Although this sounds appealing, studies show that patients still have withdrawal symptoms afterward, and the risks of anesthesia outweigh the benefits of the procedure. Outcomes are not improved with this method, and therefore it is not recommended.

How to Recognize Addiction

To fully assess any substance use disorder, a nonjudgmental approach is crucial to elicit the most accurate information from the patient. Clinicians can quickly establish rapport by sitting at eye level with the patient, maintaining eye contact, and giving full attention for a period of time. Clinicians should maintain neutrality and communicate with respect and empathy when obtaining the history.

Chronic opioid use carries a risk of overdose death, but no frank signs of toxicity are seen in any major organs; however, patients can experience impaired gonadotropin release, impaired sperm motility, menstrual irregularities, sleep disturbances, and generalized immunosuppression.

Patients can become physically dependent on opioids within 4–7 days of daily therapy, so tolerance and withdrawal are common phenomena with chronic opioid use. Box 11–3 contains DSM-5 criteria for opioid use disorder.

Box 11–3. Diagnostic Criteria for Opioid Use Disorder

A. A problematic pattern of opioid use leading to clinically significant impairment or distress, as manifested by at least two of the following, occurring within a 12-month period:

1. Opioids are often taken in larger amounts or over a longer period than was intended.
2. There is a persistent desire or unsuccessful efforts to cut down or control opioid use.
3. A great deal of time is spent in activities necessary to obtain the opioid, use the opioid, or recover from its effects.
4. Craving, or a strong desire or urge to use opioids.
5. Recurrent opioid use resulting in a failure to fulfill major role obligations at work, school, or home.
6. Continued opioid use despite having persistent or recurrent social or interpersonal problems caused or exacerbated by the effects of opioids.
7. Important social, occupational, or recreational activities are given up or reduced because of opioid use.
8. Recurrent opioid use in situations in which it is physically hazardous.
9. Continued opioid use despite knowledge of having a persistent or recurrent physical or psychological problem that is likely to have been caused or exacerbated by the substance.
10. Tolerance, as defined by either of the following:

    a. A need for markedly increased amounts of opioids to achieve intoxication or desired effect.
    b. A markedly diminished effect with continued use of the same amount of an opioid.

Note: This criterion is not considered to be met for those taking opioids solely under appropriate medical supervision.

11. Withdrawal, as manifested by either of the following:

   a. The characteristic opioid withdrawal syndrome (refer to Criteria A and B of the criteria set for opioid withdrawal).

   b. Opioids (or a closely related substance) are taken to relieve or avoid withdrawal symptoms.

   Note: This criterion is not considered to be met for those individuals taking opioids solely under appropriate medical supervision.

Specify if:
   In early remission
   In sustained remission

Specify if:
   On maintenance therapy
   In a controlled environment

Specify current severity:
   Mild: Presence of 2–3 symptoms.
   Moderate: Presence of 4–5 symptoms.
   Severe: Presence of 6 or more symptoms.

Since the 1990s, prescription opioid use has dramatically increased, resulting in a significant increase in iatrogenic addiction. Heroin use also has increased, presumably because prescription opioids are much more expensive than heroin, and patients often switch to heroin as their use increases. In the 1960s, heroin use was largely found in minority populations in urban environments, yet now heroin use is increasingly found among white men and women in their late 20s living in suburban areas (Cicero et al. 2014). Clinicians must have a high level of suspicion for opioid use disorders in patients who were not traditionally at high risk for opioid misuse.

Clinicians who suspect an opioid use disorder should consider additional screening for the following: other substance use, depression, anxiety, the safety of the patient with regard to living situation and personal relationships, and HIV and hepatitis C virus (HCV) risk factors.

What to Do About Addiction

Opioid maintenance treatment or chronic antagonist therapy always should be strongly encouraged. Outcomes for opioid detoxification are quite poor, with tremendously high relapse rates; despite its frequent practice, detoxification is unlikely to result in long-term abstinence and appears to have minimal long-term benefit. This is likely due to the protracted withdrawal syndrome that most people experience, which can last for months and even more than a year.

Pharmacological treatment for opioid use disorders includes

- Opioid maintenance
  - Methadone
  - Buprenorphine
- Antagonist therapy
  - Naltrexone (oral tablet)
  - Injectable naltrexone (monthly injection)

OPIOID MAINTENANCE

METHADONE MAINTENANCE

Methadone can be prescribed in an office or clinic setting when the indication is pain management, but it *must* be dispensed by a federally regulated opioid treatment program if the indication is an opioid use disorder. This means that individual physicians cannot prescribe methadone maintenance for a patient, and such patients must be referred to an opioid treatment program. There is one exception: an individual physician can apply to provide office-based methadone to treat opioid use disorders, but this requires approval and strict adherence to rules (Center for Substance Abuse Treatment 2005).

Methadone's long half-life of 24–36 hours allows for once-daily dosing (or even every 2 days). Titration to at least 80–100 mg/day is often necessary to eliminate cravings, provide cross-tolerance, and improve treatment retention, and many patients require even higher doses. Titration should continue as clinically indicated; dosage increases should be made in 4- to 5-day intervals to allow a steady state to be achieved. Methadone maintenance can be continued in other settings (an inpatient unit, a residential rehabilitation unit), as long as the patient's status in an opioid treatment program is verified.

Serious side effects of methadone maintenance treatment are the following:

- Hypogonadism in men
- QTc prolongation, which can progress to torsades de pointes in rare cases (Pani et al. 2013). Some opioid treatment programs perform baseline and annual electrocardiograms, but this practice is not officially recommended by the Substance Abuse and Mental Health Services Administration unless the patient has cardiac risk factors.

Minor side effects include

- Constipation
- Diaphoresis
- Drowsiness
- Decreased sexual drive

Patients often say that they heard that methadone will "rot your bones," which likely stems from patients experiencing bone pain and myalgias during withdrawal. However, there has been some evidence of an increased risk of osteopenia in patients receiving chronic opioid therapy, which may be related to hypogonadism. Patients receiving opioid maintenance may require an ongoing bowel regimen (although some studies show improved constipation after 3 years of methadone maintenance).

Methadone maintenance research has accumulated 50 years of data, and methadone maintenance is one of the best-studied interventions in all of psychiatry. It has been found to be quite safe, and along with decreasing risk of overdose death, it provides improved psychosocial adjustment, reduced criminal activity, and decreased rates of HIV and HCV infection (Ruiz and Strain 2011).

Buprenorphine Maintenance

Buprenorphine was approved in 2002 as a Schedule III medication for opioid use disorders and became the first office-based maintenance treatment available. This was made possible by DATA 2000, which allows qualified physicians to prescribe U.S. Food and Drug Administration–approved opioids from Schedules II–V for opioid use disorders in an office setting, as long as they can provide or refer patients to appropriate counseling. Physicians must complete 8 hours of training (which can be done entirely online), and they are granted a "waiver" that allows prescribing for up to 30 patients at a time. A subsequent waiver can increase this number to 100.

Buprenorphine is a partial agonist of the μ opioid receptor; it is administered sublingually and has a long half-life of 24–60 hours that can allow for less than daily dosing. See "What to Do About Withdrawal" for an induction schedule. Usual maintenance doses range from 8 to 24 mg/day. At 16 mg/day, 85%–92% of the μ opioid receptors are occupied, but some patients do not experience elimination of craving until higher doses are administered. A dose of 32 mg/day is considered the maximum, above which further benefit is not expected. Buprenorphine does not appear to have much effect on the QT interval, and although there have been reports of a mild transaminitis, the clinical significance of this is unclear. Transaminitis is more likely in patients with hepatitis, and their liver enzymes should be monitored. Minor side effects include sedation, constipation, headache, and nausea (Renner and Levounis 2010).

Because of its partial agonism, buprenorphine is equivalent to approximately 60–80 mg of methadone, so patients who require higher doses of methadone might not be good candidates for buprenorphine. Advantages of buprenorphine over methadone include

- Decreased risk of respiratory depression
- Relative safety in overdose
- Decreased sedation
- More mild withdrawal symptoms (although some patients dispute this)

Although buprenorphine alone has not been implicated in fatal overdose, some European reports have described deaths as a result of an injected combination of buprenorphine and benzodiazepines.

Buprenorphine is usually prescribed in a combination form with naloxone at a 4:1 ratio. Because naloxone is not orally bioavailable, it is activated only if the person attempts to inject the combination, in which case it would then theoretically precipitate withdrawal (and studies have shown that patients rate the "high" much more poorly when injecting the buprenorphine/naloxone combination as opposed to buprenorphine alone).

Buprenorphine lacks oral bioavailability, and it must be administered via mucosa (sublingually) or parenterally for absorption to occur. A variety of formulations are available.

Buprenorphine/naloxone is marketed in a sublingual formulation as Suboxone and, more recently, Zubsolv. A buprenorphine sublingual mono-product is marketed as Subutex (which does not contain naloxone). A buccal film version, Bunavail, contains buprenorphine/naloxone and was approved in 2014. A subdermal implant formulation, Probuphine, is still awaiting approval from the U.S. Food and Drug Administration as of early 2016, although it is expected to be available soon. This implant would deliver 6 months of buprenorphine. Finally, an intravenous/intramuscular formulation of buprenorphine, Buprenex, is indicated for moderate to severe pain but would not be used for opioid maintenance therapy.

Methadone or Buprenorphine?

While methadone has been used in treatment for over 50 years, buprenorphine has been administered for over a decade. Logistical constraints often lead to the selection of one of these treatments over the other (such as availability of methadone clinics or of buprenorphine prescribers).

It seems that all types of patients can do well with either methadone or buprenorphine. Many patients prefer the flexibility of buprenorphine, and some may describe being triggered by attending a methadone clinic daily where some patients continue to actively use drugs. Patients who require more intensive services might benefit from the higher level of structure found in a methadone clinic (although some clinics also dispense buprenorphine). As mentioned previously, fully titrated buprenorphine is only equivalent to methadone 60–80 mg, so some patients might not have cravings entirely alleviated with buprenorphine. Some studies have reported that higher-income patients tend to have more access to buprenorphine, but given its effectiveness in all socioeconomic groups (Hansen et al. 2013), it should be made available to all patients when possible. Patients with comorbid pain will experience greater relief with methadone, although it will need to be dosed three or four times a day.

Drug-Drug Interactions

Both methadone and buprenorphine are extensively metabolized. Along with some other cytochrome enzymes, cytochrome P450 (CYP) 3A4 plays a significant role in their metabolism. Drugs that induce cytochrome P450 can precipitate opioid withdrawal by accelerating metabolism. There is more data regarding interactions with methadone. For example, carbamazepine, phenobarbital, rifampin, phenytoin, and antiretrovirals such as nevirapine or efavirenz may cause the onset of withdrawal symptoms and necessitate dose adjustments of methadone. Drugs such as ciprofloxacin, fluconazole, erythromycin, and fluvoxamine can slow the metabolism of methadone and cause side effects. However, methadone can lead to increased levels of medications like zidovudine (Ries et al. 2014).

Buprenorphine also can have significant drug interactions. For example, delavirdine and atazanavir can increase buprenorphine levels. Overall, buprenorphine has fewer severe interactions compared with methadone. Clinicians should check for drug-drug interactions before starting any new medication in a patient receiving opioid maintenance treatment.

TWELVE-STEP GROUP CAVEAT

Many Alcoholics Anonymous (AA) and Narcotics Anonymous (NA) groups are opposed to opioid maintenance treatment, preferring an abstinence-only approach; some groups will not consider patients to be sober and will not allow them to "count days" while receiving opioid maintenance. It is important to be aware of this stigma in the 12-step community so that the clinician can counsel the patient on the evidence for maintenance treatment and its improved outcomes and encourage the patient to search for AA and NA groups or peers who are aware of its benefits.

ANTAGONIST THERAPY

NALTREXONE

Naltrexone is a μ opioid antagonist that blocks the effects of exogenous opioids. It can be administered at 50 mg/day or at doses of 100–150 mg three times per week. Patients must be fully detoxified before the first dose or it will induce withdrawal symptoms; this means 5–7 days for short-acting opioids and 7–10 days for long-acting opioids. Baseline liver function tests (LFTs) should be obtained, and naltrexone should not be prescribed if liver enzymes are three to five times the upper limit of normal. LFTs should be rechecked approximately 2 weeks after starting naltrexone and then periodically. Patients with hepatitis B virus or HCV are still candidates for naltrexone, but LFTs should be monitored more closely. Minor side effects include nausea and vomiting, abdominal pain, and headache; concerns about depressive symptoms and suicidality have not accumulated consistent data and remain controversial.

Naltrexone is quite effective when taken, but issues with compliance often arise. An important caveat is that patients who relapse on opioids after naltrexone use appear to have higher overdose rates, likely as a result of decreased tolerance induced by naltrexone's opioid antagonism (Ritter 2002). This phenomenon should be explained to patients, with a suggestion to "test" a much lower dose than usual if a relapse does occur.

Injectable Naltrexone

Vivitrol is a long-acting depot injection that can be given at 380 mg intramuscularly once per month and that provides a steady-state concentration of naltrexone. It improves compliance and decreases rates of relapse as compared with oral naltrexone. It is not yet known if patients also have higher overdose rates on discontinuation.

ADDITIONAL TREATMENT AND SUPPORT

Pharmacotherapy alone is rarely sufficient to treat an opioid use disorder. Patients also should be offered individual and group therapy, along with a referral to self-help groups such as AA or NA. AA and NA groups often have different "personalities" and demographic characteristics, so a patient should be encouraged to try out a few different groups if the first one does not fit. AA and NA have Web sites and hotlines that can be located via Internet search, and details about local meetings can be printed out for the patient. In a patient who is frequently relapsing, a higher level of care is warranted—such as an intensive outpatient program or inpatient rehabilitation.

Special Issues With Psychiatric Comorbidities

Comorbid psychiatric disorders are very common among patients with opioid use disorders. It is estimated that more than 40% of this patient population has a psychiatric disorder such as depression, anxiety, or bipolar disorder. The correct diagnosis can be difficult because symptoms of withdrawal and intoxication can mimic other psychiatric disorders. Taking a thorough history and observing the patient during abstinence can be helpful in making an accurate diagnosis. Untreated symptoms of anxiety or depression can lead to difficulty in engaging patients in opioid treatment, whereas concurrent treatment of other psychiatric disorders can lead to improved outcomes.

Special Issues With Medical Comorbidities

Opioid use and the route of use can be associated with many medical complications. The most common comorbid problem is infection. In addition, many opioid-dependent patients have poorly managed chronic problems such as diabetes or hypertension. Patients should be evaluated routinely for the following conditions:

- Hepatitis A, B, and C
- Syphilis and other sexually transmitted diseases
- Tuberculosis
- HIV

Educating patients about their risk for such medical conditions and providing preventive measures when appropriate are essential components of treatment; for example, patients should receive vaccination for hepatitis A and B. It is important to be aware of the infections that can be acute and potentially life-threatening:

- Endocarditis
- Soft tissue infections: abscesses and cellulitis
- Necrotizing fasciitis
- Wound botulism

Even though effective treatments are available for hepatitis C, some treatment providers might be reluctant to treat patients with an opioid use disorder. Research shows that patients who are stable on opioid maintenance treatment have good outcomes when treated for HCV, and abstinence is not a requirement. These patients benefit from coordinated care for substance abuse and their medical comorbidities.

Special Issues With Specific Populations

PREGNANCY

Opioid use during pregnancy is a challenging problem. The opioid-using pregnant patient might find it difficult to let her primary care physician or obstetrician/gynecologist know about the drug use because of stigma and legal or custody concerns, which vary by state; it can be helpful to be aware of local laws and to address this with the patient.

Risks associated with continued opioid use during pregnancy include

- Premature labor
- Intrauterine growth retardation
- Toxemia
- Antepartum and postpartum hemorrhage
- Infections

Perinatal complications include

- Low birth weight
- Increased neonatal mortality
- Increased risk of sudden infant death syndrome
- Neonatal abstinence syndrome (NAS): irritability, diarrhea, feeding problems, respiratory distress, tremors, and seizures

Long-term effects on the fetus include

- Increased inattention
- Hyperactivity
- Behavioral problems

TREATMENT OF OPIOID USE DISORDER DURING PREGNANCY

Detoxification. Detoxification is not the recommended treatment for most pregnant women because of high risk of relapse and increased risk of intrauterine death.

Methadone.   The treatment of choice for women using opioids is opioid maintenance therapy. Methadone maintenance is considered first-line treatment, and pregnant women should be referred to methadone maintenance programs. Opioid maintenance treatment at an adequate dose leads to improved maternal and neonatal outcomes. Adequate dosing of methadone prevents the fluctuations in maternal opioid levels associated with drug abuse, which result in increased stress on the fetus. Opioid maintenance is associated with decreased risk of maternal relapse and improved prenatal care, longer gestation, and higher birth weight. All opioids, including methadone, cause NAS.

Buprenorphine.   Buprenorphine represents an alternative opioid maintenance therapy. It is associated with less severe NAS. Given that it has been used to treat opioid use disorders only since 2002, it has fewer data than methadone maintenance (Jones et al. 2010).

PAIN

Management of pain in an opioid-dependent patient can be controversial and complex. Patients receiving opioid maintenance therapy have high rates of both acute and chronic pain. These patients ideally would be managed by pain management specialists. Despite, or because of, the attention that pain has received in the United States, the approach to pain management is very inconsistent, with some physicians overprescribing and others refusing to prescribe. One of the common beliefs leading to reluctance to treat pain is that usual dosing of opioid maintenance therapy will treat acute pain, which is not true. Acute pain in some of these patients could be managed by nonopioid medications and nonpharmacological therapies.

Managing Acute Pain in Patients Receiving Methadone Maintenance Treatment

- Maintain the maintenance dose of methadone, and add a short-acting opioid such as morphine, hydromorphone, or oxycodone.
- Recognize that the dose of opioid analgesic required might be higher and needed more frequently than usual because of the patient's high tolerance.

- Transition to nonopioid analgesics as soon as possible.
- Communicate with the outpatient center or provider who is treating the opioid use disorder.
- Monitor closely for both adequate pain control and for signs of possible drug abuse.
- Do not provide prescriptions with multiple refills. Patients need to be evaluated in the clinic again before providing a refill for analgesics. (Alford et al. 2006)

MANAGING ACUTE PAIN IN PATIENTS RECEIVING BUPRENORPHINE MAINTENANCE TREATMENT

- Buprenorphine blocks the analgesic effects of other opioids. If moderate to severe acute pain is anticipated for a planned surgery, hold the buprenorphine, and start a short-acting opioid. The elimination half-life of buprenorphine ranges from 24 to 60 hours, so patients may require a higher dosage of other opioid analgesics initially.
- Ensure that buprenorphine is restarted by the buprenorphine provider after the patient has stopped taking opioid medication for 12–24 hours, in order to prevent precipitation of withdrawal.
- For acute pain that is mild to moderate, consider increasing the daily dose of buprenorphine.
- Consider some other options for acute pain, including interventional procedures such as nerve blocks. (Alford et al. 2006)

MANAGING CHRONIC PAIN IN PATIENTS RECEIVING OPIOID MAINTENANCE TREATMENT

- For patients who need ongoing pain management, replace buprenorphine with methadone as the treatment for an opioid use disorder.
- Use nonpharmacological treatments such as relaxation therapy, biofeedback, cognitive-behavioral therapy, and massage before or in conjunction with opioids. Treatment of comorbid psychiatric issues is essential.
- Divide the daily maintenance methadone dosage into three-to-four-times-daily doses to better address pain, because methadone's analgesic half-life is 4–8 hours.

- Prescribe adjuvant medications for pain, including non-steroidal anti-inflammatory drugs, anticonvulsants, anti-depressants, and muscle relaxants.

Managing pain in patients who are not yet addicted to opioids includes careful risk assessment. An easy, short screen is the Opioid Risk Tool (ORT; visit www.drugabuse.gov and enter the tool name in the search feature). The ORT assesses the risk of aberrant behaviors when patients are prescribed opioid medication for chronic pain. Patients who score higher on this tool have an increased risk for opioid misuse.

ADOLESCENTS

Opioid use disorders among adolescents have been recognized as a growing problem in recent years. In large part, opioid use disorders have been linked to the increased availability of prescription opioids. Adolescents abusing opioids have high comorbid use of marijuana. Undiagnosed and untreated opioid use disorders can lead to significant morbidity and mortality. As for adults, treatment options in adolescents include counseling, medications, and the combination of the two. Unlike in the adult population, research in pharmacotherapies remains limited for adolescents (Fiellin 2008).

- Buprenorphine has been shown to be effective in managing opioid use disorders in adolescents, and it is approved by the U.S. Food and Drug Administration for patients age 16 and older.
- Methadone maintenance programs in the United States usually do not treat patients younger than 18 years. The exception is patients 16 years or older with two documented episodes of detoxification or short-term rehabilitation.
- Supportive counseling, family therapy, and close monitoring for relapse are important components of treatment.

KEY POINTS

Opioids are an indispensable tool and very effective at relieving physical (and emotional) pain, yet regular use can lead to physical dependence within days. Although opioids are medically safe at therapeutic doses, the risk of death in overdose is high because of respiratory depression.

Opioids can quickly become deadly when used recreationally. Because they are prescribed medications, a low perception of harm has driven widespread recreational misuse.

The prescription opioid epidemic, which began in the 1990s and was initiated by aggressive and unethical marketing from pharmaceutical companies, has claimed thousands of lives as a result of unintended iatrogenic addiction and subsequent overdose.

Many individuals switch to heroin when unable to obtain or afford prescription opioids, which has led to rising heroin use nationally and a demographic shift among heroin users from an inner-city minority population to white individuals living in suburban areas. Clinicians should be alert for prescription opioid misuse and addiction and routinely inquire about heroin use.

Methadone and buprenorphine are the available options for maintenance treatment of opioid use disorders. Given the startling increase in patients addicted to opioids, it is critical that more physicians become certified to prescribe buprenorphine. Oral or injectable naltrexone is an alternative pharmacological treatment for opioid use disorders.

References

Alford DP, Compton P, Samet JH: Acute pain management for patients receiving maintenance methadone or buprenorphine therapy. Ann Intern Med 144(2):127–134, 2006 16418412

American Psychiatric Association: Diagnostic and Statistical Manual of Mental Disorders, 5th Edition. Arlington, VA, American Psychiatric Association, 2013

Center for Substance Abuse Treatment: Medication-Assisted Treatment for Opioid Addiction in Opioid Treatment Programs (Treatment Improvement Protocol [TIP] Series, 43). Rockville, MD, Substance Abuse and Mental Health Services Administration, 2005

Cicero TJ, Ellis MS, Surratt HL, et al: The changing face of heroin use in the United States: a retrospective analysis of the past 50 years. JAMA Psychiatry 71(7):821–826, 2014 24871348

Fiellin DA: Treatment of adolescent opioid dependence: no quick fix. JAMA 300(17):2057–2059, 2008 18984896

Hansen HB, Siegel CE, Case BG, et al: Variation in use of buprenorphine and methadone treatment by racial, ethnic, and income characteristics of residential social areas in New York City. J Behav Health Serv Res 40(3):367–377, 2013 23702611

Jones HE, Kaltenbach K, Heil SH, et al: Neonatal abstinence syndrome after methadone or buprenorphine exposure. N Engl J Med 363(24):2320–2331, 2010 21142534

Nelson L, Lewin N, Howland MA, et al (eds): Goldfrank's Toxicologic Emergencies, 9th Edition. New York, McGraw-Hill Professional, 2010

Pani PP, Trogu E, Maremmani I, et al: QTc interval screening for cardiac risk in methadone treatment of opioid dependence. Cochrane Database Syst Rev 6:CD008939, 2013 23787716

Renner JR, Levounis P: Handbook of Office-Based Buprenorphine Treatment of Opioid Dependence. Washington, DC, American Psychiatric Publishing, 2010

Ries RK, Fiellin DA, Miller SC, et al (eds): The ASAM Principles of Addiction Medicine, 5th Edition. Philadelphia, PA, Lippincott Williams & Wilkins, 2014

Ritter AJ: Naltrexone in the treatment of heroin dependence: relationship with depression and risk of overdose. Aust N Z J Psychiatry 36(2):224–228, 2002 11982544

Ruiz P, Strain E (eds): Lowinson and Ruiz's Substance Abuse: A Comprehensive Textbook, 5th Edition. Philadelphia, PA, Lippincott Williams & Wilkins, 2011

Substance Abuse and Mental Health Services Administration: Results from the 2013 National Survey on Drug Use and Health: Summary of National Findings, NSDUH Series H-48, HHS Publ No SMA 14-4863. Rockville, MD, Substance Abuse and Mental Health Services Administration, 2014. Available at: http://www.samhsa.gov/data/sites/default/files/NSDUHresultsPDFWHTML2013/Web/NSDUHresults2013.pdf. Accessed February 29, 2016.

Van Zee A: The promotion and marketing of oxycontin: commercial triumph, public health tragedy. Am J Public Health 99(2):221–227, 2009 18799767

Wesson DR, Ling W: The Clinical Opiate Withdrawal Scale (COWS). J Psychoactive Drugs 35(2):253–259, 2003 12924748. Available at: https://www.drugabuse.gov/sites/default/files/files/ClinicalOpiateWithdrawalScale.pdf. Accessed March 7, 2016.

CHAPTER 12

Stimulants

DOUGLAS OPLER, M.D.

SHAOJIE HAN, M.D., M.S.

STIMULANT drugs of abuse and addiction include cocaine, amphetamines, "bath salts," piperazines, and ephedra.

- **Cocaine:** Illicit cocaine is marketed in two forms, both as the salt, cocaine hydrochloride, which can be administered intranasally or subcutaneously because of its water solubility, and as the freebase crystalline form known as "crack," which has a lower melting point that allows it to be smoked. Cocaine use grew to epidemic proportions in North American cities in the 1980s and peaked around 1985, with Colombia being a major source of supply. Today, most cocaine arrives in the southwestern United States via the Mexican border and is often heavily adulterated with a variety of substances, including local anesthetics, caffeine, sugars, other stimulants, contaminants, and even the antihelminthic agent levamisole. Levamisole-contaminated cocaine can result in unfortunate adverse effects, including cutaneous vasculitis.
- **Amphetamines:** Amphetamine is placed under Schedule II in the United States because of its abuse potential, although this scheduling still allows it to be prescribed. Indications include attention-deficit/hyperactivity disorder (ADHD) and narcolepsy. Similarly, formulations of methamphetamine continue to have indications for both ADHD and obesity.

    Street names for methamphetamine include "crystal meth," "crank," and "ice." Methamphetamine is synthesized in underground laboratories. Use has been declining in the United States since the beginning of the twenty-first century, when restrictions were placed on availability of the precursor compound pseudoephedrine. Imports through Mexico have begun to replace American manufacture. Chemical variations on amphetamine include 3,4-methylenedioxymethamphetamine (MDMA, also known as "Ecstasy").

- **"Bath salts":** More properly called *synthetic cathinones*, "bath salts" are synthetic chemical derivatives of cathinone, the active chemical in the plant khat, *Catha edulis*. Cathinone itself has been a Schedule I drug since 1988, and the first synthetic cathinone gained Schedule I status in the United States in 1993. The nickname "bath salts" was given because they are frequently marketed under that guise in an attempt to avoid legal scrutiny. Packages of "bath salts" are sold under brands such as Ivory Wave, Bliss, Energy, White Lightning, Meow, and MCAT. They can be found in online stores, gas stations, and head shops and bear the false disclaimer "Not intended for human consumption." The most common synthetic cathinone in the United States is 3,4-methylenedioxypyrovalinone (MDPV). Other "bath salts" in circulation include mephedrone, methylone, and α-pyrrolidinopentiophenone (α-PVP). (Rosenbaum et al. 2012)

- **Piperazines:** The piperazines are another group of emerging stimulant drugs. The drug benzylpiperazine was originally used as an antihelminthic compound but was later found to have amphetamine-like properties. Benzylpiperazine and its derivatives have subsequently become a new addition to the pharmacopoeia of illicitly abused stimulants. Although they share a small chemical moiety with the antipsychotics of the same name, the stimulant piperazines are otherwise structurally and functionally dissimilar from the class of typical phenothiazine antipsychotics also known as piperazines. (Rosenbaum et al. 2012)

- **Ephedra:** Like coca (the botanical source of cocaine) and khat (the botanical source of cathinone), ephedra is a botanical stimulant. Derived from the plant Ephedraceae, it was used in Chinese medicine for at least 5,000 years. More recently, ephedra has been abused for its stimulant effect and beliefs that it can help achieve weight loss, enhance athletic performance, and increase libido. Cases of adverse effects and death from overdose have been reported. Ephedra was banned for sale in the United States by the U.S. Food and Drug Administration (FDA) in 2004. However, ephedra is still advertised for illegal sale via the Internet.

Pharmacology

The effects of the stimulants are primarily mediated through activity on the monoamine neurotransmitters: dopamine, norepinephrine, and serotonin (Table 12–1). Stimulants act through one of two basic mechanisms, being either transporter blockers or transporter substrates (Table 12–2). Monoamine transporters are molecules present on the neuronal cell membrane, which normally function to remove extracellular monoamines from the synaptic cleft and return them to the intracellular space. In the presence of a transporter blocker, this normal function is impaired, thereby preventing the transporter from returning neurotransmitters to the intracellular space. As a result, extracellular monoamine concentrations build up. Transporter substrates, on the other hand, are taken up by the monoamine transporter and actually reverse the function of the monoamine transporter, causing it to release monoamines from the intracellular space into the synaptic cleft. In doing so, they also deplete vesicular stores of monoamines. Both transporter blockers and transporter substrates lead to increased synaptic monoamine concentrations.

Different stimulants vary in how much they alter the function of any particular monoamine transporter (see Table 12–1). Cocaine, the amphetamines, methylphenidate, and MDPV all affect reuptake of both dopamine and norepinephrine, whereas phentermine and ephedrine preferentially affect reuptake of norepinephrine. Cocaine, methylone, and mephedrone also have serotonergic properties.

In addition to both direct and centrally mediated cardiovascular and stimulating effects via the sympathetic nervous system, the effects of stimulants are mediated via the mesocorticolimbic dopamine pathway. This pathway projects from an area in the midbrain called the ventral tegmental area, where the cell bodies of dopaminergic neurons reside. The axons of these neurons have synapses in the prefrontal cortex, the nucleus accumbens, and the amygdala. When the dopamine transporters responsible for removing dopamine from these synapses are prevented from functioning under the influence of stimulants, dopamine concentrations in the

Stimulants

TABLE 12–1. Major monoamine transporter effects of stimulants

Stimulant	Dopamine	Norepinephrine	Serotonin
Amphetamine	+	+	
Cocaine	+	+	+
Ephedrine		+	
3,4-Methylenedioxypyrovalinone (MDPV)	+	+	
Mephedrone	+	+	+
Methylone	+	+	+
Methylphenidate	+	+	
Phentermine		+	

Note. "+" indicates that the listed stimulant interferes with the reuptake transporter of the indicated monoamine neurotransmitter.

TABLE 12–2. Stimulants classified by mechanism

Mechanism	Stimulants
Transporter blocker	Cocaine, methylphenidate, 3,4-methylenedioxypyrovalinone (MDPV)
Transporter substrate	Amphetamines, ephedrine, phentermine, methylone, mephedrone

synapses rise, leading to increased binding to dopamine receptors in these locations. Increased dopamine receptor binding in the nucleus accumbens is experienced as a rewarding and euphoric high by the user.

Although multiple types of dopamine receptors exist and modulate various functions, the dopamine type 1 (D_1) receptor in the nucleus accumbens is thought to be important in the actions of stimulants. Activation of the D_1 receptor in the nucleus accumbens inhibits the action of the globus pallidus on motor nuclei. The globus pallidus normally functions to decrease motor nuclei activity. Therefore, inhibition of globus pallidus function by dopaminergic activity in the nucleus accumbens ultimately disinhibits motor nuclei, thereby contributing to the stimulating effects of these drugs.

The route of administration of stimulants alters their time to effect. When smoked, stimulants reach the brain within 8 seconds, rapidly leading to clinical effects. Peak concentrations in the brain occur following intravenous use within 4–7 minutes, whereas oral or intranasal stimulants can take as long as 30–45 minutes to take effect. Smoked and intravenous stimulant use also has a greater effect on the user because of greater bioavailability than oral or intranasal use.

TOXICOLOGY

Cocaine and amphetamines are metabolized primarily by the liver and eliminated via the urine. As a result, amphetamines and cocaine metabolites can be detected via urine screening. Standard urine toxicology assays for stimulants vary in the length of time that they are able to detect different stimulants. Amphetamine and methamphetamine can be detected for up to 2 days, whereas cocaine metabolites can be detected for 3–4 days. Standard toxicology screens do not test for other stimulant drugs. However, many commercial laboratory vendors do offer expanded drug screens for commonly used synthetic cathinones. Illicit manufacturers of emerging drugs of abuse, however, are frequently marketing new structural variations on compounds, which may not be detected by available toxicology panels. Various medications can potentially produce false-positive amphetamine screens, notably including

- Amantadine
- Bupropion
- Chlorpromazine
- Desipramine
- Labetalol
- Phenylephrine
- Promethazine
- Pseudoephedrine
- Ranitidine
- Selegiline
- Thioridazine
- Trazodone
- Trimipramine

Legal stimulants prescribed under medical supervision and taken as directed (e.g., for ADHD) also can result in a positive amphetamine screen. As a result, a detailed medication history should be taken when interpreting a positive amphetamine toxicology result. Amphetamine elimination is enhanced when urine is acidified, and is impaired when urine pH is raised. In order to manipulate this, amphetamine users will sometimes take high doses of sodium bicarbonate to prolong amphetamine effects and avoid detection on urine drug screens.

How to Recognize Intoxication

Stimulants cause pupillary dilation in intoxication. Box 12–1 contains DSM-5 criteria for stimulant intoxication (American Psychiatric Association 2013).

Box 12–1.   Diagnostic Criteria for Stimulant
                    Intoxication

A. Recent use of an amphetamine-type substance, cocaine, or other stimulant.

B. Clinically significant problematic behavioral or psychological changes (e.g., euphoria or affective blunting; changes in sociability; hypervigilance; interpersonal sensitivity; anxiety, tension, or anger; stereotyped behaviors; impaired judgment) that developed during, or shortly after, use of a stimulant.

C. Two (or more) of the following signs or symptoms, developing during, or shortly after, stimulant use:

1. Tachycardia or bradycardia.
2. Pupillary dilation.
3. Elevated or lowered blood pressure.
4. Perspiration or chills.
5. Nausea or vomiting.
6. Evidence of weight loss.
7. Psychomotor agitation or retardation.
8. Muscular weakness, respiratory depression, chest pain, or cardiac arrhythmias.
9. Confusion, seizures, dyskinesias, dystonias, or coma.

D. The signs or symptoms are not attributable to another medical condition and are not better explained by another mental disorder, including intoxication with another substance.

Specify **the specific intoxicant** (i.e., amphetamine-type substance, cocaine, or other stimulant).

Specify if:
With perceptual disturbances

Mood alterations with stimulant use may vary and can include

- Anxiety
- Euphoria
- Dysphoria
- Irritability
- Relaxation

At low doses, effects of stimulants may include

- Increased energy
- Increased alertness

- Self-confidence
- Sociability
- Decreased need for sleep
- Decreased appetite
- Increased libido

At higher doses, effects of stimulants may include

- Increasing activation and excitement
- Insomnia
- Anorexia
- Restlessness
- Panic attacks
- Confusion and delirium
- Psychosis, including delusions, hallucinations, grandiosity, and paranoia
- Repetitive, purposeless behaviors known as "punding," which can include skin picking and disassembly of mechanical objects

Hallucinations can be of various types, but tactile hallucinations are often prominent with stimulant use. Psychosis is more commonly seen with the amphetamines than with cocaine but can occur with either. After chronic amphetamine use, psychosis may become persistent, although such persistence is not usually seen with chronic cocaine use in the absence of a primary psychotic disorder. The psychiatric syndrome seen with stimulant intoxication can be difficult to distinguish from a manic or psychotic episode as might be seen in bipolar disorder, schizophrenia, or schizoaffective disorder. If symptoms persist for 24 hours after drug use, a psychiatric rather than substance-induced etiology of the syndrome should be considered. A longitudinal history and observation during a period of abstinence can be helpful in unclear cases. Stimulant-induced psychosis generally resolves after several days of discontinuation, although more persistent syndromes of psychosis have been described.

Stimulant intoxication is potentially dangerous. Diverse medical complications of use can include

- Tremor
- Dyskinesia
- Tachycardia

- Hypertension
- Myocardial infarction
- Palpitations
- Arrhythmias
- Seizures
- Stroke
- Hyperthermia
- Rhabdomyolysis
- Delirium

Chronic stimulant use may lead to a host of other sequelae affecting multiple organ systems as well.

OBTAINING THE HISTORY

The clinician should determine stimulant use (type, amount, method, last use) and any comorbid drug or alcohol use. He or she should inquire about newer drugs of abuse, including questions about "bath salts," and collect collateral information from family, friends, and medical records, as available.

What to Do About Intoxication

Assessment of stimulant intoxication should include medical and psychiatric evaluation, including physical examination and monitoring of vital signs. Laboratory testing should include urine toxicology, but standard toxicology panels do not include newer drugs of abuse. Specialized expanded panels are available from commercial vendors to test for some of the more common synthetic stimulants, but these are not yet widely available in hospital laboratories.

If the patient is experiencing psychotic symptoms, treatment with antipsychotics may be necessary. Electrocardiogram and QTc interval should be checked, and the potential effect of QTc-prolonging medications, including antipsychotics, should be taken into account. However, if hyperthermia, agitation, or rhabdomyolysis is present, creatinine phosphokinase levels should be measured, and high doses of benzodiazepines may be a safer treatment option than neuroleptics. Supportive and symptom-specific treatments will depend on the patient's individual presentation. β-Blockers generally should be avoided given the potential vasoconstrictive effect of unopposed alpha activity.

How to Recognize Withdrawal

Stimulants cause pupillary contraction in withdrawal. Following a binge, individuals may experience diverse symptoms, such as

- Fatigue
- Depression
- Anhedonia
- Anxiety
- Impaired concentration
- Increased appetite
- Increased dreaming
- Increased need for sleep
- Intense cravings
- Suicidal ideation

Rarely, myocardial ischemia has been described. Withdrawal may last for several days after discontinuation of the drug or may persist for several weeks. Box 12–2 contains DSM-5 criteria for stimulant withdrawal.

Box 12–2.   Diagnostic Criteria for Stimulant Withdrawal

A. Cessation of (or reduction in) prolonged amphetamine-type substance, cocaine, or other stimulant use.

B. Dysphoric mood and two (or more) of the following physiological changes, developing within a few hours to several days after Criterion A:

  1. Fatigue.
  2. Vivid, unpleasant dreams.
  3. Insomnia or hypersomnia.
  4. Increased appetite.
  5. Psychomotor retardation or agitation.

C. The signs or symptoms in Criterion B cause clinically significant distress or impairment in social, occupational, or other important areas of functioning.

D. The signs or symptoms are not attributable to another medical condition and are not better explained by another mental disorder, including intoxication or withdrawal from another substance.

Specify **the specific substance that causes the withdrawal syndrome** (i.e., amphetamine-type substance, cocaine, or other stimulant).

What to Do About Withdrawal

Stimulant withdrawal typically can be treated supportively and usually does not require hospitalization. Although myocardial ischemia has been described, medical intervention is rarely required for stimulant withdrawal. The patient's mental status and suicide risk should be assessed, and suicidal ideation may necessitate hospitalization. If the patient presents a risk of danger to self, psychiatric admission and antidepressant medication may be necessary. Fatigue is best treated with rest. Behavioral interventions should be used to manage the increased risk of relapse during this period.

How to Recognize Addiction

Comprehensive assessment of a stimulant use disorder requires a full history that examines biological, psychological, and social aspects of use. An empathetic and nonjudgmental approach should be maintained when acquiring the history in order to maximize the accuracy of the information obtained, to maintain rapport, and to solicit compliance with any necessary interventions. In addition to an in-depth history of drug use, social and forensic history should be thoroughly explored. The motivations for seeking treatment and any tendency to deny substance use can both heavily affect the presentation of the illness. In clinical settings, users may be prone to exaggerate discomforts and dysphoria during withdrawal in order to obtain treatment, but in other contexts, they may be more likely to minimize the significance of use and underreport amounts of use to avoid punitive and legal consequences. Given this, collateral information from sources other than patients may be of great value.

Box 12–3 contains DSM-5 criteria for stimulant use disorder. As for stimulant intoxication and stimulant withdrawal, DSM-5 criteria for stimulant use disorder require that the specific stimulant be included in the diagnosis name (e.g., "cocaine use disorder"), whether an amphetamine-type substance, cocaine, or other stimulant.

Box 12–3. Diagnostic Criteria for Stimulant Use Disorder

A. A pattern of amphetamine-type substance, cocaine, or other stimulant use leading to clinically significant impairment or distress, as manifested by at least two of the following, occurring within a 12-month period:

1. The stimulant is often taken in larger amounts or over a longer period than was intended.
2. There is a persistent desire or unsuccessful efforts to cut down or control stimulant use.
3. A great deal of time is spent in activities necessary to obtain the stimulant, use the stimulant, or recover from its effects.
4. Craving, or a strong desire or urge to use the stimulant.
5. Recurrent stimulant use resulting in a failure to fulfill major role obligations at work, school, or home.
6. Continued stimulant use despite having persistent or recurrent social or interpersonal problems caused or exacerbated by the effects of the stimulant.
7. Important social, occupational, or recreational activities are given up or reduced because of stimulant use.
8. Recurrent stimulant use in situations in which it is physically hazardous.
9. Stimulant use is continued despite knowledge of having a persistent or recurrent physical or psychological problem that is likely to have been caused or exacerbated by the stimulant.
10. Tolerance, as defined by either of the following:
    a. A need for markedly increased amounts of the stimulant to achieve intoxication or desired effect.
    b. A markedly diminished effect with continued use of the same amount of the stimulant.

    Note: This criterion is not considered to be met for those taking stimulant medications solely under appropriate medical supervision, such as medications for attention-deficit/hyperactivity disorder or narcolepsy.
11. Withdrawal, as manifested by either of the following:
    a. The characteristic withdrawal syndrome for the stimulant (refer to Criteria A and B of the criteria set for stimulant withdrawal).
    b. The stimulant (or a closely related substance) is taken to relieve or avoid withdrawal symptoms.

    Note: This criterion is not considered to be met for those taking stimulant medications solely under appropriate medical supervision, such as medications for attention-deficit/hyperactivity disorder or narcolepsy.

Specify if:
  In early remission
  In sustained remission
Specify if:
  In a controlled environment
Specify current severity:
  Mild: Presence of 2–3 symptoms.
  Moderate: Presence of 4–5 symptoms.
  Severe: Presence of 6 or more symptoms.

Stimulant use disorders can develop as rapidly as 1 week, although they often take longer to develop and can lead to significant impairment or distress. Tolerance and withdrawal are common in individuals with stimulant use disorders and can be helpful features suggestive of addiction. However, when stimulants are used under medical supervision for treatment of an appropriate indication, tolerance and withdrawal without additional features of addiction should not be considered indicative of addiction.

Collateral informants may suspect stimulant use when changes in behavior start to manifest, including hyperactivity, elated mood, or violent behaviors. Personality and mood changes may develop over time. Alternatively, discovery of drug paraphernalia may alert family members to a patient's stimulant use. Other potential signs of use in the history may include

- Dishonest or secretive behaviors
- Neglect of social responsibilities
- Lack of personal hygiene
- Mood swings
- Dysphoria and psychosis
- Selling personal belongings
- Stealing to fund drug use

Physical signs of use observed by the clinician or reported by the family may assist in identifying addiction, such as

- Dilated pupils
- Hypersensitivity to light
- Chronic nasal inflammation from intranasal insufflation
- Needle marks caused by injection

Prescribers and pharmacists can play important roles in identifying prescription stimulant addiction. Incorporation of screening for addiction into regular medical visits is essential to allow for early identification and intervention. Prescribers of stimulants should be aware of any rapid increases in dosage, early refill requests, or potential "doctor shopping" behaviors. The prescriber should discuss with the patient some guidelines on appropriate medication use. The patient should be alerted that any future red flags or inappropriate use of medications will require discontinuation of the medication. Such discussions should be held before any problems occur rather than waiting until after problematic patterns of use start to present themselves. Collaborative care and communication among a patient's different providers can be useful, as can prescription drug monitoring programs. Such programs require physicians and pharmacists to log filled prescriptions into a state database, which can help to identify prescription stimulant addiction when such databases are available.

Surreptitious underreporting of use is frequent in both teenage and adult stimulant users. One study showed that drug testing of hair samples was 52 times more likely to identify cocaine use compared with self-reported use by teenagers (Delaney-Black et al. 2010). In the same study, self-report of cocaine use was compared to drug testing results of cocaine use in the parents of the same teenagers. Testing demonstrated that the adult parents of the teenagers were also likely to be underreporting cocaine use. Testing of the parents was 6.5 times more likely to reveal cocaine use than the parents' self-reports. Urine testing, which is more widely available, is even less likely to detect stimulant use within its shorter window of detection. However, urine tests in emergency departments have particularly high yields in screening of high-risk groups for stimulant use. When stimulant use is suspected, random unannounced urine testing is essential for identifying use.

What to Do About Addiction

BEHAVIORAL INTERVENTIONS

Behavioral interventions are an important component of treatment for stimulant use disorders. They can be implemented alone, combined with one another, or combined with pharmacotherapy. They are nonspecific for any one stimulant addiction and flexible in treating different stages of stimulant addiction. Common behavioral interventions for stimulant addiction include the following (Kosten et al. 2012):

- *Motivational interviewing:* A way to prepare patients for life changes by facilitating the patient's own sense of autonomy to choose healthy behaviors. It can be of particular use with resistant or ambivalent patients who are not yet committed to change and do not yet feel ready for substance addiction treatment.
- *Contingency management:* An approach that seeks to decrease the frequency of drug use by pairing substance use or abstinence with a series of consequences contingent on the behavior. For example, some predetermined period of abstinence on the part of the patient may be tied to a reinforcing consequence to support this abstinence. Reinforcers can take many forms, including money, vouchers exchangeable for goods or services, or access to television privileges in a residential setting. Contingency management has been found to be helpful in reducing cocaine use, but treatment effects may not be maintained after contingency management ceases.
- *Cognitive-behavioral therapy (CBT):* A form of collaborative psychotherapy that (in the case of stimulant use disorders) seeks to decrease drug use by examining distorted thoughts and problematic behaviors related to use and teaching the patient how to replace such thoughts and behaviors with more accurate thoughts and more functional behaviors. Patients are taught to monitor and recognize precipitants of use and to cope with cravings. CBT has been found to be particularly effective in the treatment of stimulant use disorders when combined with medication and contingency management.
- *Group counseling:* Various group counseling formats are available to stimulant users and their friends or families. Narcotics Anonymous, Cocaine Anonymous, Crystal Meth Anonymous, and other 12-step programs emphasize relinquishing control to a higher power, such as God or the group. CBT-oriented group counseling shares some of the structure of 12-step approaches, but in contrast to the traditional 12-step approach of relinquishing control, CBT-oriented group treatments emphasize gaining self-control through the use of CBT techniques. Psychody-

namic group counseling can provide a safe environment for patients to explore their personal vulnerabilities related to addiction.

PHARMACOTHERAPY

So far, the FDA has not approved any medications for the treatment of stimulant use disorder. Research into pharmacotherapy for stimulant use disorder has faced the challenging question of which neurotransmitter systems should be targeted for treatment. Newly discovered knowledge in neurobiology has yet to translate into effective pharmacotherapies. Most research on pharmacological treatments has focused on cocaine use disorder. These results may apply to the treatment of other stimulant use disorders as well.

Agonist therapy seeks to use stimulants themselves to treat stimulant use disorder, much like methadone is successfully used in the treatment of opioid addiction. Agonist approaches that have been studied include

- *Amphetamines:* Small clinical trials showed that dextroamphetamine administration reduced cocaine and methamphetamine use or craving (Forray and Sofuoglu 2014). Its long-term safety and efficacy remain to be determined.
- *Modafinil:* Initial clinical trials were promising, but larger trials have not shown effectiveness in treatment of cocaine use.
- *Bupropion:* A dopamine and norepinephrine reuptake inhibitor itself, bupropion is used in the treatment of depression and ADHD and in smoking cessation; it has little abuse potential. When combined with contingency management, bupropion significantly improved treatment outcomes in cocaine use disorder.
- *Disulfiram:* Increases synaptic levels of dopamine by inhibiting enzymatic degradation. It is effective in reducing cocaine use in clinical trials. However, disulfiram may result in cocaine accumulation, especially under the influence of alcohol.
- *Desipramine:* When combined with CBT, desipramine improved treatment retention and abstinence in depressed cocaine users.

No other antidepressants or mood stabilizers have proved reliably efficacious in reducing cocaine use when prescribed alone. Data on other medications have borne mixed or preliminary results, although these medications may be promising future candidate treatments pending confirmatory studies. These include

- Medications that target noradrenergic systems, including lofexidine, carvedilol, guanfacine, and prazosin
- Medications targeting the γ-aminobutyric acid system, including vigabatrin, topiramate, and baclofen
- N-Acetylcysteine, which has effects on glutamate activity
- Galantamine, an acetylcholinesterase inhibitor that improved both cognition and abstinence in cocaine users
- TA-CD, a cocaine vaccine that induces antibody formation
- Progesterone in cocaine-dependent women, which may attenuate cravings for and subjective effects of stimulants

Special Issues With Psychiatric Comorbidities

Comorbid psychiatric disorders are very common among stimulant users and often include

- Schizophrenia
- Bipolar disorder
- ADHD
- Antisocial personality disorder
- Posttraumatic stress disorder
- Major depressive disorder
- Other substance use disorders

Comorbid bipolar disorder, antisocial personality disorder, alcohol use disorder, and opioid use disorder are all associated with an increased severity of cocaine use disorder, whereas cannabis use disorder is associated with a decreased severity of cocaine use disorder.

Hypotheses for the high rates of comorbidity have been proposed, one being that individuals with primary psychiatric disorders attempt to self-medicate with stimulants to relieve negative emotions or to combat the sedative effects of psychotropic medications. A second hypothesis is that the underlying pathology of the altered brain circuitry and behavioral abnormalities in primary psychiatric disorders also predisposes patients toward impulsivity, cognitive deficits, or other factors that promote stimulant addiction.

Providers may have concerns about prescription of stimulant medications, but appropriate prescription treatment of ADHD does not appear to lead to increased substance misuse by patients. However, it may be prudent for clinicians to seek specialist psychiatric input in such cases to assist with diagnosis and the formulation of a prescription treatment plan.

Special Issues With Medical Comorbidities

RESPIRATORY COMORBIDITIES

Patients with preexisting pulmonary disease may experience worsening of symptoms with either intranasal cocaine use or crack cocaine use. This may include exacerbation of

- Asthma and chronic obstructive pulmonary disease
- Pulmonary edema
- Interstitial pneumonitis
- Eosinophilic lung disease
- Pulmonary vascular disease
- Pneumothorax
- Pneumomediastinum

In addition to worsening preexisting comorbidities, stimulant use can result in new respiratory problems in users. Nasal congestion is the most common medical complication associated with intranasal cocaine and amphetamine use. Inflammation, bleeding, ulceration, and perforation of the nasal septum also may occur. Crack cocaine use can also lead to respiratory complications, such as

- Cough
- Increased sputum production
- Wheezing
- Dyspnea
- Hemoptysis
- Chest pain
- Burn injuries of the upper airways
- Tracheal stenosis
- Pulmonary fibrosis

- Pulmonary hypertension
- Pulmonary hemorrhage

Intravenous cocaine and amphetamines may cause pulmonary damage via pulmonary microemboli from fillers and adulterants.

CARDIOVASCULAR COMORBIDITIES

Because cocaine and amphetamine stimulate the sympathetic nervous system, the risk of adverse cardiovascular events is markedly increased in users. Adverse cardiovascular effects may include

- Chest pain
- Atherosclerosis
- Hypertension
- Acute coronary syndrome and myocardial infarction
- Aortic dissection
- Cardiomyopathy
- Myocarditis
- Left ventricular hypertrophy
- Sudden cardiac death

Some amphetamine derivatives (e.g., fenfluramine) are also known to potentially induce valvular heart disease. In treating cardiovascular adverse events resulting from stimulant use, note that β-blockers should not be used without adequate α-blockade, or unopposed vasoconstrictive effects can ensue.

OTHER MEDICAL COMORBIDITIES

Cocaine can have a range of effects on other organ systems as well (Table 12–3), which can lead to additional medical comorbidities, such as

- Dental caries
- Gingivitis
- Seizures
- Renal failure
- Rhabdomyolysis
- Stroke
- Autoimmune diseases
- Connective tissue diseases

TABLE 12–3. Adverse effects of cocaine by organ system

Organ system	Adverse effects
Cardiac	Chest pain, tachycardia, hypertension, myocardial infarction, coronary atherosclerosis, cardiac arrhythmias, myocardial fibrosis, myocarditis, cardiomyopathy, left ventricular hypertrophy
Dental	Bruxism, gingival ulceration, erosion of dental enamel, caries, tooth loss
Dermatological	Cutaneous vasculitis (from either cocaine itself or levamisole adulterants)
Ear, nose, and throat	Rhinitis, perforation of nasal septum, nasal collapse, sinusitis
Endocrine	Prolactin abnormalities, increased risk of diabetic ketoacidosis
Gastrointestinal	Decreased gastric motility, gastric and duodenal ulcers, intestinal infarction, gastric perforation, intestinal perforation, viral hepatitis (transmitted during injection use)
Male reproductive	Erectile dysfunction, delayed ejaculation, priapism, reduced sperm count, impaired sperm motility
Musculoskeletal	Rhabdomyolysis, muscular vasculitis
Neurological	Tremor, cognitive impairment, dyskinesia, seizure, stroke, cerebrovascular atherosclerosis

TABLE 12–3. Adverse effects of cocaine by organ system *(continued)*

Organ system	Adverse effects
Obstetrical/ gynecological	Irregular menses, premature rupture of membranes, placental abruption, placenta previa, decreased infant head circumference, decreased infant size
Ophthalmological	Corneal ulcers (with crack cocaine use)
Psychiatric	Dysphoria, euphoria, anxiety, panic attacks, irritability, paranoia, psychosis, hallucinations, grandiosity, impaired judgment, restlessness, anorexia
Pulmonary	Cough, dyspnea, hemoptysis, wheezing, pulmonary edema, pulmonary hemorrhage, pneumothorax, pneumomediastinum, burns to the upper airway, interstitial pneumonitis, bronchiolitis obliterans
Renal	Ischemia, infarction, renal tubular obstruction (from rhabdomyolysis)

Special Issues With Specific Populations

CHILDREN AND ADOLESCENTS

Increased prescription of stimulant medications to children and adolescents has raised concerns about diversion and the abuse potential of stimulant medications. Nonmedical use of stimulants has been reported in young adults and college students at a rate from 5% to 35%. Although such users often initially use stimulants to improve attention and cognition in order to boost academic performance, the euphoric and dependence-forming properties of the medications can contribute to future abuse and addiction.

PREGNANCY AND BREAST-FEEDING

Most stimulants are classified in pregnancy as Category C by the FDA, although the risks of newer stimulants are unknown, and adulterants in street stimulants may present additional dangers. Potential risks of stimulant medications in pregnant users include

- Premature rupture of membranes
- Placental abruption
- Placenta previa

Effects on the infant may include decreased head circumference and decreased birth weight. Appropriate use of prescribed stimulants under medical supervision, however, is not thought to have any significant effects on the infant.

KEY POINTS

Behavioral interventions form the core treatment modalities for stimulant use disorders and include motivational interviewing, contingency management, cognitive-behavioral therapy, and group counseling. Research on pharmacotherapy for stimulant use disorders has yielded largely mixed or preliminary results.

The psychiatric syndrome that results from stimulant intoxication can be difficult to distinguish from a manic or psychotic episode as might be seen in bipolar disorder or primary psychotic disorders, but if symptoms persist for 24 hours after stimulant use, a primary psychiatric rather than substance-induced etiology of the syndrome should be considered.

Prescription stimulants have indications in various disorders, including attention-deficit/hyperactivity disorder, narcolepsy, and obesity. When the stimulants are taken as prescribed under appropriate medical supervision, the risk of addiction is low. However, the prescriber should discuss guidelines for proper use with the patient at the time of medication initiation and be alert for any potential signs of misuse, including running out of medications early, frequently losing prescriptions, rapidly increasing dose, "doctor shopping" behavior, and obtaining stimulants from multiple providers. Collaborative care and prescription drug monitoring programs can be useful in identifying problematic patterns of use.

References

American Psychiatric Association: Diagnostic and Statistical Manual of Mental Disorders, 5th Edition. Arlington, VA, American Psychiatric Association, 2013

Delaney-Black V, Chiodo LM, Hannigan JH, et al: Just say "I don't": lack of concordance between teen report and biological measures of drug use. Pediatrics 126(5):887–893, 2010 20974792

Forray A, Sofuoglu M: Future pharmacological treatments for substance use disorders. Br J Clin Pharmacol 77(2):382–400, 2014 23039267

Kosten TR, Newton TF, De La Garza R II, et al (eds): Cocaine and Methamphetamine Dependence: Advances in Treatment. Washington, DC, American Psychiatric Publishing, 2012

Rosenbaum CD, Carreiro SP, Babu KM: Here today, gone tomorrow... and back again? A review of herbal marijuana alternatives (K2, Spice), synthetic cathinones (bath salts), kratom, Salvia divinorum, methoxetamine, and piperazines. J Med Toxicol 8(1):15–32, 2012 22271566

CHAPTER 13

Tobacco

TIMOTHY KOEHLER BRENNAN, M.D., M.P.H.

ANNIE LÉVESQUE, M.D.

CAYLIN RILEY, B.S.

TOBACCO is available in a variety of formulations (smoke, snuff, chew, dip), but the overwhelming majority of tobacco is smoked via commercially produced cigarettes. The financial costs associated with tobacco use are staggering and amount to more than $300 billion per year in the United States ($170 billion in direct health care costs, $156 billion in lost productivity).

Although tobacco is used throughout the world, use is increasing at the highest rates in the developing world. It is expected that by 2030, 80% of the annual deaths from tobacco will occur in developing countries. The overall prevalence of smoking has steadily declined in the United States, from 42% in 1965 to less than 20% in 2014 (Centers for Disease Control and Prevention 2015). Previously, there was a large gender gap among smokers (men>women), but as of 2013, men were only 5% more likely to smoke than women.

Cigarette smoking is now the leading cause of preventable mortality and responsible for more than 5 million annual deaths worldwide. About one-half of all tobacco users will die from a tobacco-related disease, with most causes being

- Cardiovascular disease
- Pulmonary cancers
- Chronic obstructive pulmonary disease

Pharmacology

When an individual smokes a cigarette, nicotine enters the central nervous system (CNS) within approximately 10 seconds. Although nicotine is responsible for the release of a variety of neuroactive hormones, the most important activity of nicotine is as a nicotinic acetylcholine receptor agonist that produces a stimulant-like effect in the CNS. Nicotine enhances concentration, alertness, and arousal. Nicotine also causes mild analgesia and anxiolysis and extends the positive effects of dopamine, which can increase the sensitivity in the brain's reward pathway. In commonly used recreational smoking doses, nicotine's primary effect is that of a stimulant, with higher doses producing more sedation and analgesia.

How to Recognize Intoxication

Tobacco intoxication is not a diagnosable syndrome in DSM-5 (American Psychiatric Association 2013). Nevertheless, patients who smoke a sudden and large amount of cigarettes may certainly feel unwell. Supportive care is the mainstay of treatment.

What to Do About Intoxication

Patients who have used an amount of tobacco far in excess of their typical consumption pattern may experience an acute nicotine or tobacco intoxication. Supportive care with hydration, antiemetics as needed, anxiolytics as needed, and reassurance are the mainstays of tobacco intoxication management.

How to Recognize Withdrawal

Tobacco withdrawal syndrome is likely related to deficiencies in dopamine levels. It requires patients first to be daily users of tobacco for several weeks. The syndrome is characterized as a group of symptoms that occur on abrupt cessation of or dramatic decrease in consumption of nicotine (typically within 24 hours). Box 13–1 contains DSM-5 criteria for tobacco withdrawal (American Psychiatric Association 2013).

Box 13-1. Diagnostic Criteria for Tobacco Withdrawal

A. Daily use of tobacco for at least several weeks.

B. Abrupt cessation of tobacco use, or reduction in the amount of tobacco used, followed within 24 hours by four (or more) of the following signs or symptoms:

1. Irritability, frustration, or anger.
2. Anxiety.
3. Difficulty concentrating.
4. Increased appetite.
5. Restlessness.
6. Depressed mood.
7. Insomnia.

C. The signs or symptoms in Criterion B cause clinically significant distress or impairment in social, occupational, or other important areas of functioning.

D. The signs or symptoms are not attributable to another medical condition and are not better explained by another mental disorder, including intoxication or withdrawal from another substance.

What to Do About Withdrawal

Tobacco or nicotine withdrawal can be easily treated with nicotine replacement therapy (NRT), which is available via

- Nicotine lozenges
- Nicotine gum
- Nicotine patches
- Nicotine nasal sprays
- Nicotine inhalers

Tobacco users who are admitted to the hospital often have tobacco or nicotine withdrawal syndrome. These complaints may be overtly expressed by the patients themselves or be more subtle and unstated. NRT is widely available in most hospital formularies and can be easily used in prewritten hospital order sets. Furthermore, inpatient hospitalization can be a uniquely motivating period for tobacco users interested in learning more about smoking cessation. Information and literature about cessation strategies should be freely available to these patients.

How to Recognize Addiction

Tobacco addiction—or tobacco use disorder, as it is known in DSM-5—is often self-diagnosed by patients and does not require any type of laboratory work, imaging, or tissue pathology. DSM-5 defines *tobacco use disorder* as a problematic pattern of tobacco use leading to clinically significant impairment or distress, as manifested by at least 2 of 11 signs and symptoms, occurring within a 12-month period (Box 13–2). Despite these clinical criteria, most patients with tobacco use disorder simply self-disclose as "smokers" and are diagnosed on the basis of their self-report alone.

Box 13–2.   Diagnostic Criteria for Tobacco Use Disorder

A. A problematic pattern of tobacco use leading to clinically significant impairment or distress, as manifested by at least two of the following, occurring within a 12-month period:

1. Tobacco is often taken in larger amounts or over a longer period than was intended.
2. There is a persistent desire or unsuccessful efforts to cut down or control tobacco use.
3. A great deal of time is spent in activities necessary to obtain or use tobacco.
4. Craving, or a strong desire or urge to use tobacco.
5. Recurrent tobacco use resulting in a failure to fulfill major role obligations at work, school, or home (e.g., interference with work).
6. Continued tobacco use despite having persistent or recurrent social or interpersonal problems caused or exacerbated by the effects of tobacco (e.g., arguments with others about tobacco use).
7. Important social, occupational, or recreational activities are given up or reduced because of tobacco use.
8. Recurrent tobacco use in situations in which it is physically hazardous (e.g., smoking in bed).
9. Tobacco use is continued despite knowledge of having a persistent or recurrent physical or psychological problem that is likely to have been caused or exacerbated by tobacco.
10. Tolerance, as defined by either of the following:
    a. A need for markedly increased amounts of tobacco to achieve the desired effect.

For the nonforthcoming patient, a variety of physical stigmata can indicate tobacco addiction. These traits include

- Tobacco stains on the fingertips
- Discolorations or deterioration of intraoral mucosa
- Smelling of cigarettes

More subtle clinical signs may include

- Repeated aerodigestive complaints, such as chronic cough
- Gastroesophageal reflux disease
- Low exercise tolerance
- Erectile dysfunction

Many physicians characterize tobacco use by calculating cigarette "pack-years." Pack-years are calculated by multiplying the number of cigarette packs smoked per day by the number of years that the patient has smoked cigarettes. Each pack has 20 cigarettes. For example, a smoker who has smoked a half-pack of cigarettes per day for 10 years would have a 5-pack-year history of smoking ($0.5 \times 10 = 5$).

As a quick screen for tobacco use disorder, the provider can simply begin by asking whether the patient has smoked cigarettes in the past year. Anyone revealing that he or she smokes cigarettes with any sort of regularity should be further screened with the Fagerström test (Table 13–1). The scores from this tool can be used both to guide cessation treatment and to counsel patients on the severity of their tobacco use.

TABLE 13–1. Fagerström Test for Nicotine Dependence

1. How soon after waking do you smoke your first cigarette?

   Within 5 minutes (3); 5–30 minutes (2); 31–60 minutes (1)

2. Do you find it difficult to refrain from smoking in places where it is forbidden?

   Yes (1); No (0)

3. Which cigarette would you hate to give up?

   First one in morning (1); Any other (0)

4. How many cigarettes a day do you smoke?

   31+ (3); 21–30 (2); 11–20 (1); 10 or less (0)

5. Do you smoke more frequently in the morning?

   Yes (1); No (0)

6. Do you smoke even if you are sick in bed most of the day?

   Yes (1); No (0)

Scoring
*1–2 = low dependence; 3–4 = low to moderate dependence;
5–7 = moderate dependence; 8+ = high dependence*

Source. Heatherton et al. 1991.

What to Do About Addiction

Because tobacco is responsible for a profound amount of morbidity and mortality, tremendous research has focused on tobacco addiction. Combating tobacco addiction occurs at both the public health and the individual patient level.

Public health interventions include

- Antismoking advertisements
- Increased taxes on commercial sale of tobacco products

- Age restrictions on tobacco purchasing
- Limits on the ability to smoke cigarettes in publicly accessible locations

ADVERTISING

Historically, tobacco advertisements were widely used in almost all forms of media, but current U.S. legislation severely restricts pro-tobacco advertisements. In 1970, Congress passed the Public Health Cigarette Smoking Act, which served to ban the advertisement of cigarettes on both television and radio. The Family Smoking Prevention and Tobacco Control Act (2009) went even further to restrict the advertisement of tobacco by prohibiting sponsorship of music, sports, and certain cultural events. While legislators continue their efforts to restrict pro-tobacco advertising, the public health community has created specific antismoking campaigns. These campaigns are designed by antismoking consumer groups, public health charities (especially cancer charities), and government agencies.

INCREASING TAXES

Both state and federal legislators have worked to increase the taxes on cigarette sales. These efforts are typically lauded by public health workers because many studies have shown that cigarette purchasing rates decline when cigarette prices are raised.

AGE RESTRICTIONS

A component of the Family Smoking Prevention and Tobacco Control Act (2009) gave the U.S. Food and Drug Administration (FDA) complete control over the regulation of tobacco products. In 2010, the FDA created regulations designed to limit the accessibility of tobacco products to children. It is currently illegal in the United States for tobacco products to be sold to anyone younger than 18. Some states and certain counties have increased the age required to purchase tobacco products to older than 18. Tobacco products must be sold via face-to-face transactions and not online or via vending machines, further limiting the ability of underage children to purchase tobacco.

PUBLIC SMOKING BANS

Concerns about the dangers of environmental tobacco smoke and efforts to decrease individual smoking rates have resulted in a variety of public smoking bans across municipalities and states. Many studies have documented the success of public smoking bans for public health, as well as individual health. Some businesses (typically in the restaurant and hospitality industries) have protested that these bans might harm their sales, but research has largely shown that public smoking bans have very little effect on businesses.

INDIVIDUAL ADDICTION TREATMENT

NON-MEDICATION-BASED TOBACCO CESSATION

Various tobacco cessation programs are used by individuals, counselors, and public health departments. Some of these strategies involve a predetermined quit date, with a preemptive gradual decline in the amount of tobacco consumed, as well as self-imposed limits on the accessibility of tobacco in the patient's immediate environment. Other strategies involve one-on-one counseling or self-help-based coaches, many of which are now available via text messaging or social media platforms. Tobacco cessation support groups are modeled on group therapy modalities for other conditions. In addition, it has become increasingly common for states to set up a version of a "QuitLine," which is a toll-free number that individuals can call to speak with a counselor, coordinate a quit attempt, and, in some cases, receive free NRT via mail (all through state funding).

MEDICATION-BASED TOBACCO CESSATION

A number of smoking cessation pharmacotherapies are available, as summarized in Table 13–2 and discussed further in this section.

Nicotine replacement therapy. NRT involves the delivery of nicotine in methods other than via the tobacco plant. NRT is available as

- Lozenges
- Gum
- Transdermal patches
- Nasal sprays
- Inhalers

TABLE 13–2. Smoking cessation pharmacotherapies

Drug	Route	Dosage	Duration of treatment
Nicotine lozenge	Lozenge	1 lozenge every 1–2 h (weeks 1–6) 1 lozenge every 2–4 h (weeks 7–9) 1 lozenge every 4–8 h (weeks 10–12)	12 weeks
Nicotine gum	Chew	<25 cigarettes/day=2-mg strength ≥25 cigarettes/day=4-mg strength Up to 24 pieces/day	12 weeks
Nicotine patch	Transdermal	>10 cigarettes/day=21 mg/day×6 weeks then 14 mg/day×2 weeks then 7 mg/day×2 weeks ≤10 cigarettes/day=14 mg/day×6 weeks then 7 mg/day×2 weeks	10 weeks or 8 weeks
Nicotine spray	Nasal spray	1–2 sprays/h (maximum=10/h and 40/day)	Not established
Nicotine inhaler	Inhaled	6–16 cartridges/day	3 months then 6- to 12-week wean
Bupropion	Oral	150 mg/day×3 days 150 mg twice a day×7–12 weeks	7–12 weeks

TABLE 13–2. Smoking cessation pharmacotherapies *(continued)*

Drug	Route	Dosage	Duration of treatment
Varenicline	Oral	0.5 mg/day (days 1–3) 0.5 mg twice a day (days 4–7) 1 mg twice a day×11 weeks	12 weeks or 24 weeks

Tobacco addiction often includes both physical addiction to nicotine and a learned behavioral addiction to the act of tobacco consumption. NRT products can help combat tobacco addiction on both of these fronts. Repeated trials have shown that NRT can cause a twofold increase in cessation rates when compared with placebo. Combination NRT (ideally with a patch plus either gum, spray, or inhaler) has been found in meta-analyses to be more effective than single-product therapy (Cahill et al. 2013).

Initial doses of NRT are based on the number of cigarettes smoked daily. NRT doses should be gradually tapered as nicotine withdrawal symptoms subside. NRT is generally recommended for 2–3 months after smoking cessation. Some patients will gradually decrease the amount that they are smoking while concurrently using NRT. This is believed to be acceptable as well.

Bupropion. Bupropion is an aminoketone atypical antidepressant that has an FDA indication for depression, seasonal affective disorder, and smoking cessation, although the exact mechanism of action is only partially understood. Current prescribing guidelines for bupropion recommend that patients begin bupropion 7–10 days before tobacco cessation because 5–7 days are needed for bupropion to reach steady-state blood levels. The treatment should be continued for 7–12 weeks after smoking cessation. Bupropion can reduce nicotine cravings and raise the chances of quitting smoking successfully. Bupropion has been found to outperform placebo in smoking cessation. Bupropion should not be prescribed to patients with seizure disorders because it can lower the seizure threshold. Furthermore, patients who could be potentially prone to seizures, such as those with anorexia or bulimia, brain lesions, or alcohol and sedative withdrawal, should not be given bupropion.

Varenicline. Varenicline is a nicotinic receptor partial agonist that has an FDA indication for smoking cessation. Varenicline stimulates nicotine receptors more weakly than nicotine and reduces cravings for nicotine, as well as reduces the ability of nicotine to bind to the nicotine receptors via competitive binding. A Cochrane systematic review (Cahill et al. 2013) concluded that varenicline improved successful quitting likelihood by two- to threefold relative to nonmedication cessation attempts and also found that it is more efficacious than bupropion but not any superior to NRT. Varenicline should be started 1 week before the cessation date and if successful after 12 weeks, it should be continued for 24 weeks of total treatment. Varenicline carries an FDA black box warning regarding suicidality and use is cautioned in people with cardiovascular disease.

Failure of pharmacotherapy. Patients who fail one type of pharmacotherapy should first be evaluated for proper use of the original pharmacotherapy. If the initial use attempt was done correctly, then patients should be offered alternative or combination pharmacotherapy for a future quit attempt.

Special Issues With Psychiatric Comorbidities

Rates of tobacco use disorder are significantly higher among patients who have mental illnesses compared with the general population. Those rates are particularly high in patients diagnosed with schizophrenia, in whom the prevalence of cigarette smoking is estimated between 70% and 90%. Unfortunately, smokers with comorbid psychiatric illnesses remain undertreated and have a poor response to traditional smoking cessation interventions. Barriers to treatment initiation include beliefs that smoking cessation may exacerbate the patient's psychiatric symptoms. However, negative psychiatric outcomes following smoking cessation have not been reported with consistency and should not be a reason to delay intervention. Further studies must be conducted to assess more effective treatments for nicotine dependence aimed at this specific population. As for now, patients with mental health disorders should be questioned systematically about cigarette smoking, and general approaches to tobacco cessation should be applied. The following considerations should be taken into account regarding pharmacological interventions:

- Both varenicline and bupropion can cause neuropsychiatric symptoms. Close monitoring is recommended when initiating treatment in patients with a psychiatric history.
- The use of varenicline is not recommended in patients with unstable mental disorders or with a history of suicidal ideation.
- Bupropion should be used cautiously in patients who are already taking one or more antidepressant medications.

Despite such concerns, the most effective treatment modality should be offered when indicated, and fear of neuropsychiatric consequences should not lead to undertreatment of nicotine dependence among patients with mental disorders.

Special Issues With Medical Comorbidities

Tobacco smoking is the leading cause of preventable death worldwide. It is estimated that individuals who smoke during their entire adulthood have a decreased life expectancy by about 10 years compared with nonsmokers (World Health Organization 2011). Mortality and morbidity associated with cigarette smoking are mostly mediated through the occurrence of the following health conditions.

CANCER

Smoking is a risk factor for the development of numerous cancers: oral cavity, pharynx, larynx, bladder, esophagus, cervix, kidney, lung, pancreas, stomach, liver, bowel, and acute myeloid leukemia. The number of years of use, the number of cigarettes smoked per day, and the depth of inhalation all influence the impact of carcinogenic effects of cigarettes.

CARDIOVASCULAR DISEASES

Cigarette smoking is a major risk factor of cardiovascular disease. Nicotine use can lead to coronary vasoconstriction, increased hypercoagulability, dyslipidemia, and endothelial dysfunction—all of which contribute to hypertension, myocardial infarctions, and strokes.

RESPIRATORY ILLNESSES

ASTHMA

Airway irritation caused by cigarette smoking can exacerbate respiratory symptoms in asthmatic patients. Smoking cessation and decreasing environmental tobacco smoke are key elements in the treatment of asthma.

CHRONIC OBSTRUCTIVE PULMONARY DISEASE

Cigarette smoking can lead to chronic obstructive pulmonary disease. Smoking cessation is associated with improved lung function, reduced chronic cough and mucus production, and reduced chronic obstructive pulmonary disease–related mortality.

OTHER CONDITIONS

Cigarette smoking is also a risk factor for the following conditions:

- Type 2 diabetes
- Osteoporosis
- Cataracts and macular degeneration
- Early menopause
- Erectile dysfunction
- Gastric and duodenal ulcer disease
- Skin aging
- Periodontal disease

RECOMMENDATION

Many of the risks associated with smoking can be completely or partially reversed following sustained cessation. This supports the importance of encouraging every patient to quit, including those who have already developed health consequences of tobacco use.

Special Issues With Specific Populations

PREGNANCY

In the United States, 11% of pregnant women report smoking cigarettes during the last 3 months of pregnancy (Tong et al. 2013). This number is concerning given the well-documented adverse outcomes associated with tobacco use in pregnancy. Mechanisms involved in such complications are not completely understood and may include decreased oxygen supply, direct toxicity, and sympathetic activation. Importantly, sustained exposure to environmental tobacco smoke in pregnancy can lead to similar consequences (Leonardi-Bee et al. 2011).

Risks associated with tobacco smoking in pregnancy include

- Spontaneous pregnancy loss
- Placental abruption
- Ectopic pregnancy

- Placenta previa
- Preterm premature rupture of membranes
- Preterm labor and delivery

Perinatal complications include

- Low birth weight
- Sudden infant death syndrome

The effects of tobacco smoking on breast-feeding include

- Decreased milk volume production
- Lower milk fat concentration
- Shorter duration of lactation

TREATMENT OF TOBACCO USE DISORDER DURING PREGNANCY

Pregnancy is the moment at which women are more likely to quit smoking. The ideal timing to initiate interventions is before conception, and clinicians should discuss smoking cessation with every woman considering pregnancy. When preconception cessation is not achieved, prenatal care visits provide a unique platform to implement interventions, allowing for sustained counseling and support. Although data are lacking regarding the efficacy and safety of pharmacological treatments for smoking cessation in pregnancy, expert committees support their use for patients who failed to quit with psychosocial treatments, considering that the risks associated with smoking continuation exceed those of taking medications. Both NRT and bupropion are acceptable first-line options. Potential adverse effects of the medication should be discussed with patients before initiating treatment:

- *NRT (gum, nasal spray, and lozenges: Class C; patch: Class D):* NRT can cause sympathetic activation and vasoactive effects, increasing the risk of hypertension and placental abruption. No evidence indicates that teratogenic effects are associated with NRT. Pregnant women have increased nicotine metabolism and may require higher doses.
- *Bupropion (Class C):* Most available data suggest low risk in pregnancy; however, one study reported increased risk of miscarriage following the use of bupropion during the first trimester. Another study (Thyagarajan et al. 2012)

suggested increased prevalence of left ventricular out-flow tract obstruction among fetuses exposed to bupropion in the first trimester, although the small number of cases led to unclear conclusions on this association.

- *Varenicline (Class C):* This medication is not recommended in pregnancy given insufficient data regarding treatment safety and efficacy in this population.

ADOLESCENTS

Adolescent smoking is a significant public health concern. Considering that about 90% of adults with tobacco use disorder began smoking before age 18, early intervention is particularly important in preventing prolonged use and future health consequences. Exploring the various incentives and barriers to quitting should be part of counseling with teenagers. Adolescents may consider financial aspects, improved general health, and athletic capacity as incentives to quit, but they frequently express concerns about weight gain and discomfort from withdrawal.

Efficacy and safety of pharmacological treatments are not well established for adolescent populations; therefore, psychosocial interventions are generally recommended as a first-line approach. However, when sustained abstinence fails to be achieved with a nonpharmacological approach, NRT can be used in combination with psychosocial interventions to maximize the chances of success. In the United States, NRT is sold over the counter for adults, but it requires a prescription for use in children younger than age 18. Data are insufficient regarding the use of bupropion and varenicline in adolescents, and therefore these pharmacotherapies are not recommended in this population.

KEY POINTS

Tobacco addiction is the most likely cause of preventable mortality in the world.

All clinicians should be knowledgeable about tobacco cessation strategies.

Nicotine replacement therapy and pharmacotherapy are widely available and easy-to-use interventions for patients who wish to stop using tobacco.

References

American Psychiatric Association: Diagnostic and Statistical Manual of Mental Disorders, 5th Edition. Arlington, VA, American Psychiatric Association, 2013

Cahill K, Stevens S, Perera R, Lancaster T: Pharmacological interventions for smoking cessation: an overview and network meta-analysis. Cochrane Database Syst Rev 2013 May 31;5:CD009329. doi: 10.1002/14651858.CD009329.pub2

Centers for Disease Control and Prevention: Cigarette Smoking in the United States. December 14, 2015. Available at: http://www.cdc.gov/tobacco/campaign/tips/resources/data/cigarette-smoking-in-united-states.html. Accessed March 4, 2016.

Family Smoking Prevention and Tobacco Control Act: Pub. L. No. 111-31 [H.R. 1256]; 123 Stat. 1776. June 22, 2009. Available at: http://www.fda.gov/TobaccoProducts/GuidanceCompliance-RegulatoryInformation/ucm246129.htm. Accessed March 4, 2016.

Heatherton TF, Kozlowski LT, Frecker RC, Fagerström KO: The Fagerström Test for Nicotine Dependence: a revision of the Fagerström Tolerance Questionnaire. Br J Addict 86(9):1119–1127, 1991 1932883

Leonardi-Bee J, Britton J, Venn A: Secondhand smoke and adverse fetal outcomes in nonsmoking pregnant women: a meta-analysis. Pediatrics 127(4):734–741, 2011 21382949

Thyagarajan V, Robin Clifford C, Wurst KE, et al: Bupropion therapy in pregnancy and the occurrence of cardiovascular malformations in infants. Pharmacoepidemiol Drug Saf 21(11):1240–1242, 2012 23109236

Tong VT, Dietz PM, Morrow B, et al: Trends in smoking before, during, and after pregnancy—Pregnancy Risk Assessment Monitoring System, United States, 40 sites, 2000–2010. MMWR Surveill Summ 62(6):1–19, 2013 24196750

World Health Organization: WHO report on the global tobacco epidemic, 2011: warning about the dangers of tobacco. Geneva, World Health Organization, 2011. Available at: http://www.who.int/tobacco/global_report/2011/en. Accessed March 4, 2016.

CHAPTER 14

Behavioral Addictions

Focus on Gambling Disorder

TIMOTHY FONG, M.D.

CAN a person become addicted to a behavior such as gambling or sex? Is this an actual psychiatric condition or a convenient way to explain deviant or immoral behavior? Over the last 25 years, scientific evidence has emerged to show that behavioral addictions, also known as non-substance-related disorders, have similar biological, psychological, and social risk factors and pathology to chemical addictions.

Clinicians are often faced with presenting complaints of excessive gambling, hypersexual behaviors, or inability to stop playing video games. Although universal acceptance of the pathophysiology and diagnostic criteria of behavioral addictions remains to be established, the prevalence and clinical effect of these conditions are significant. Historically, these patterns of behaviors have been classified as obsessive-compulsive spectrum disorders, impulse-control disorders, or by-products of mood disorders.

Providers need to accurately discern and be able to assess when excessive behavioral patterns require psychiatric intervention or whether presenting problems fall within the realm of normative behavior. As with most disorders, classification of a diagnostic threshold is made by gathering as much information about the presenting problem from as many reliable sources as possible and then differentiating these symptoms from more parsimonious explanations of the chief complaint.

In the case of behavioral addictions, it is important that patients be evaluated in the context of several other factors, including the extent to which their behavior

- Disrupts personal, family, social, or vocational pursuits
- Causes significant personal distress to self or others
- Has risk or potential for significant physical or emotional harm to self or others
- Is uncontrollable or resistant to change (e.g., patient feels out of control or unable to reduce or change the behavior)
- Is not better accounted for by an alternative psychiatric diagnosis

At this time, only one behavioral addiction is formally categorized in DSM-5 (American Psychiatric Association 2013): gambling disorder. Behavioral addictions such as gambling disorder can present in a variety of subtle and deceptive patterns. Because of the intense shame, guilt, and embarrassment felt by patients, it may fall to providers to use screening tools and more in-depth interviewing techniques to uncover the extent of these behaviors. Identifying when the line is crossed from recreation or habit to psychopathology relies on understanding current diagnostic criteria and consideration of cultural, ethnic, and local community standards. Individuals are also likely to cross back and forth over this line between pathology and habit, further clouding the provider's opinions of diagnosis—therefore, tracking and monitoring these symptoms over time are critical to establishing patterns of use and documenting ongoing consequences. Treatment for gambling disorder is emerging slowly, and treatment outcomes for these conditions appear to be similar to those for other addictive disorders. This chapter will review the prevalence, clinical presentation, and management principles of gambling disorder.

Gambling

Gambling can be defined as risking something of value (usually money) on the outcome of an event decided by chance with the hopes of winning a reward (also, usually money). In the United States, gambling is a widely available and acceptable form of entertainment and recreation. Legalized gambling is present in all but two states (Hawaii and Utah), and nearly 65% of the general population report placing a wager in the last year. Legal gambling revenue exceeds the combined earnings from movies, sporting events, and amusements parks.

Clinicians are encouraged to stay in tune with the types of gambling offered in their state and to follow along as emerging gambling trends occur. The main opportunities to gamble in the United States include land-based casinos, Internet gambling, and nonregulated gambling. Newer forms of gambling include online fantasy sports games. These online services are legal to operate and participate in. Typically, players wager on daily fantasy sports games and compete against other players for the best performance of their online teams. In summary, gambling has never been more available or accessible at any other time in U.S. history.

The vast majority of people who gamble regularly do so without incurring long-lasting harm or adverse consequences. However, approximately 1%–2% of the general population meet criteria for gambling disorder, which means that it is as prevalent as schizophrenia or bipolar disorder. Gambling addiction was first recognized in DSM-III (American Psychiatric Association 1980) with scientific criteria and was classified as pathological gambling in the "Impulse-Control Disorders" section. As more research has been conducted, scientific evidence has pointed problem and pathological gambling toward the addictions model. Currently, DSM-5 recognizes pathological gambling as an addictive disorder and places it in the "Substance-Related and Addictive Disorders" section with a new name, gambling disorder.

Pharmacology

Although no substances are ingested, the act of gambling has been shown to affect levels of natural neurochemicals—chiefly dopamine, norepinephrine, cortisol, and serotonin. Dopamine is released in the brain, in the same regions where it is released with use of alcohol and drugs of abuse, in response to situations involving the prospects of obtaining a reward (increased attention and motivation) and earning or winning a reward (experiencing pleasure). Evidence shows that persons with gambling disorder have alterations in functioning in all of these neurotransmitter systems, raising the question of how these changes and alterations occur in the first place.

How to Recognize Intoxication

The concept of intoxication from gambling has not been formally recognized, but many patients describe a dissociative, numb feeling while gambling. Casino employees are trained to recognize the signs of problem gambling and impaired judgment that will lead to continued gambling, including behaviors such as extended (beyond 12 hours) gambling sessions, hostility, dramatic outbursts, or visible bouts of anger and frustration. Gamblers report subjective responses similar to those caused by drugs of abuse in anticipation of and while gambling. Emotional reports of euphoria, calmness, feelings of peace, sexual arousal, and overall wellness have been described by individuals who are gambling.

A medical definition of *intoxication* is an abnormal state that is essentially a poisoning. The state of excessive or prolonged gambling can certainly occur, with case reports of persons gambling nonstop, without breaks, for 24–36 hours. These states are likely to result in significant decline in physical and mental health functioning, and the medical effects are similar to those of any prolonged activity—sleep deprivation, impaired judgment, muscle breakdown, and prolonged state of adrenergic tone. Clinicians can very easily miss signs of recent and excessive gambling behaviors because no single pathognomonic sign of gambling intoxication exists. A much more common scenario involves drug or alcohol intoxication that fuels and drives ongoing gambling. Substances of abuse affect gambling by diminishing the meaning of losses and accentuating the desire to pursue wins by increasing risk-taking and impulsive behaviors.

What to Do About Intoxication

Given the nature of a gambling binge, its effects, any comorbid conditions, and differential diagnoses, refer to the sections "How to Recognize Addiction" and "What to Do About Addiction" later in this chapter for discussion of how to address this addictive disorder.

How to Recognize Withdrawal

A withdrawal syndrome is associated with gambling disorder. Gambling withdrawal is associated with increased urges or cravings to gamble, restlessness, anxiety, and irritability when unable to gamble. Clinically significant withdrawal can be distinguished from normal reactions to missing gambling when the symptoms impair functioning or rise to the level of significant distress. This period of time, which can last several days, has been associated with a high likelihood of relapse and return to gambling.

What to Do About Withdrawal

The gambling withdrawal state is self-limited and, in most cases, resolves on its own in 3–5 days. Supportive medications such as benzodiazepines for acute and short-term management of the subjective distress associated with withdrawal may be helpful, but prescribers must be cautious to avoid exacerbating other addictive disorders and potentially disinhibiting an already impulsive population. Left untreated or unaddressed, ongoing withdrawal symptoms from gambling are likely to lead to relapse, ongoing distress, or both. Brief psychotherapy such as motivational interviewing, supportive therapy, and psychoeducational therapy are likely to help facilitate discussion that will raise awareness in the patient, families, and additional therapists about how to manage gambling withdrawal.

A protracted abstinence syndrome also may emerge with gambling disorder and has been shown to occur several months after individuals have been free from gambling. Individuals have reported ongoing gambling urges and emotional reactions to gambling advertisements or reminders of past gambling episodes (such as driving past the casino or receiving casino mailings), which have been shown to trigger preoccupations with gambling and a possible return to gambling. Providers are reminded to continually ask about these symptoms to reduce the likelihood of relapse, and to consider that nonspecific psychiatric symptoms may be related to gambling.

How to Recognize Addiction

Gambling disorder can be a *hidden addiction* in that the consequences of gambling can be kept secret from close friends and family members. Clinicians are urged to discuss and identify patterns of problem gambling and can do so with short screening tools. Two examples of these are the Lie/Bet Questionnaire (Johnson et al. 1997; available at: http://www.ncrg.org/sites/default/files/uploads/docs/monographs/liebet.pdf) and the Brief Biosocial Gambling Screen (Gebauer et al. 2010; available at: http://www.ncrg.org/resources/brief-biosocial-gambling-screen). The Lie/Bet Questionnaire asks two questions selected from the DSM-IV (American Psychiatric Association 1994) criteria for pathological gambling because they were identified as the best predictors of gambling disorder. The Brief Biosocial Gambling Screen asks three questions about gambling behavior over the past 12 months.

Diagnostic interviews that use DSM-5 criteria for gambling disorder (Box 14–1; American Psychiatric Association 2013) will allow clinicians to differentiate recreational gambling from gambling disorder. In regard to making a clear gambling disorder diagnosis, gambling that occurs secondary to dopamine agonists or gambling that occurs during the course of a manic episode must be ruled out as well. Severity of gambling disorder is established in terms of number of DSM-5 criteria met—mild gambling disorder is equivalent to four to five criteria met, moderate gambling disorder is six to seven criteria met, and severe gambling disorder is eight to nine criteria met.

Box 14–1. Diagnostic Criteria for Gambling Disorder

A. Persistent and recurrent problematic gambling behavior leading to clinically significant impairment or distress, as indicated by the individual exhibiting four (or more) of the following in a 12-month period:

1. Needs to gamble with increasing amounts of money in order to achieve the desired excitement.
2. Is restless or irritable when attempting to cut down or stop gambling.
3. Has made repeated unsuccessful efforts to control, cut back, or stop gambling.
4. Is often preoccupied with gambling (e.g., having persistent thoughts of reliving past gambling experiences, handicapping or planning the next venture, thinking of ways to get money with which to gamble).
5. Often gambles when feeling distressed (e.g., helpless, guilty, anxious, depressed).
6. After losing money gambling, often returns another day to get even ("chasing" one's losses).
7. Lies to conceal the extent of involvement with gambling.
8. Has jeopardized or lost a significant relationship, job, or educational or career opportunity because of gambling.
9. Relies on others to provide money to relieve desperate financial situations caused by gambling.

B. The gambling behavior is not better explained by a manic episode.

Specify if:
Episodic
Persistent

Specify if:
In early remission
In sustained remission

Specify current severity:
Mild: 4–5 criteria met.
Moderate: 6–7 criteria met.
Severe: 8–9 criteria met.

During the diagnostic interview and assessment, clinicians should focus on obtaining information about the individual's gambling behavior, including how often (frequency), how long (duration), and how much (amount) he or she gambles relative to what he or she can afford to lose. Focusing on identifying clear, negative consequences is a must. These consequences may include, but may not be limited to, financial problems (e.g., bankruptcy, lost job, sizable debt), legal problems (e.g., crime, arrests), relational problems (e.g., divorce, domestic violence, child abuse), and health problems (e.g., increased stress, sleep disturbances).

A summary of activities clinicians should do to recognize and assess gambling disorder include the following:

- Use a gambling disorder screen with every patient at intake and annually.
- Collect urine toxicology to identify other sources of problematic gambling behaviors.
- Obtain collateral information to verify and clarify the extent of self-reported gambling activities.
- Ask about all forms of gambling, including stocks, real estate investments, and lottery; ask about settings where patients gamble.

What to Do About Addiction

Treatment for gambling disorders, like all addictive disorders, is best approached with a biopsychosocial treatment approach and with an integrated or multidisciplinary team creating an individualized treatment plan. No one strategy has been shown to be superior to others, which can create challenges and opportunities for clinicians in developing an effective treatment plan.

BIOLOGICAL TREATMENTS

No U.S. Food and Drug Administration (FDA)–approved medications are available for the treatment of gambling disorders. Several medications, from the addiction model, have been investigated as treatments to target the urges and cravings related to gambling. To date, medications from several different classes, including antidepressants (selective serotonin reuptake inhibitors, bupropion), anticonvulsants (lithium, valproic acid, topiramate), and antipsychotics (olanzapine, quetiapine), have been examined but have uncertain effectiveness (Achab and Khazaal 2011). The most promising data have been with opioid antagonists, naltrexone and nalmefene, which have been shown in double-blind, placebo-controlled trials to diminish gambling urges and behaviors (Hodgins et al. 2011). Additional agents that have been investigated but whose efficacy and effectiveness have not been established outside of clinical trials include N-acetylcysteine, varenicline, and acamprosate (Grant et al. 2010).

Treatment experiences with gambling disorder patients point to medicating co-occurring disorders, such as depression or anxiety disorders, that may be exacerbating or fueling gambling behavior. Clinicians are cautioned about the use of benzodiazepines, dopamine agonists, opioids, and stimulants for gambling disorder in patients without attention-deficit/hyperactivity disorder (ADHD), because overuse of these medications may result in ongoing gambling or exacerbation of underlying, co-occurring conditions.

PSYCHOLOGICAL TREATMENTS

Most psychological treatment research studies have examined the effect of behavioral, cognitive, and cognitive-behavioral therapy and motivational interviewing for gambling disorder. At this time, no one psychological treatment can be stated to have the most efficacy with patients. Even brief motivational interventions and self-help techniques have been shown to make a significant difference in reducing gambling problems.

Most psychological treatments are delivered in an office-based setting with either a gambling treatment or substance abuse specialist. The modality chosen for treatment might vary depending on symptomatology, background experience of the provider, and level of interest and psychological-mindedness of the patient. Length of time in treatment should be considered, given that no set number of treatments has been determined to be ideal, but treatment should proceed for at least 6–12 months after full recovery and development of a strong support system.

Once a gambling disorder is identified, clinicians should consider referring patients to a gambling treatment program or specialist if one is locally accessible. Many states have no-cost treatments available, which, in conjunction with a primary care provider or mental health provider, can significantly improve treatment outcomes. Residential and intensive outpatient programs for gambling disorder are available, but enrollment should be reserved for patients who require significant structure and who are at risk for self-injurious behavior or whose continued gambling could cause permanent and severe damage to the family or society.

SOCIAL TREATMENTS

The mainstay of social treatments for gambling disorder is building up of social capital to promote wellness, support, and community. Gamblers Anonymous is a mutual self-help group for gambling disorder patterned after Alcoholics Anonymous. Gamblers Anonymous is free and offers support for family members in the form of Gam-Anon. Gamblers Anonymous has been shown to be most effective when gamblers attend for an extended time, obtain a sponsor, and have a commitment at meetings (such as setting up chairs or other organizational tasks). Other social treatment modalities include sober companions, life coaches, and personal assistants to help transition patients into a lifestyle of recovery by ensuring compliance with treatment team recommendations, providing transport to recovery meetings, and monitoring behaviors. No formal studies have examined the utility of these types of social recovery activities, but they are currently used by gambling treatment programs.

Treatment principles for gambling disorder are similar to treatment principles used for substance use disorders, principally focusing on engaging the patient into a lifestyle of recovery and self-care that includes managing stress, engaging in physical activity, increasing social capital, and promoting healthy sleep hygiene.

Special Issues With Psychiatric Comorbidities

Co-occurring psychiatric disorders are the rule, not the exception, with gambling disorder; the most common conditions are major depressive disorder, bipolar disorder, and substance use disorders. ADHD and personality disorders (namely borderline, narcissistic, and antisocial personality disorders) are also seen in those with gambling disorder. When treating gambling disorder, it is crucial and pivotal that the underlying and co-occurring disorder be addressed. Left untreated or unrecognized, any co-occurring disorder will likely worsen the gambling itself because gambling is the coping factor to deal with emotional stress.

Because co-occurring substance use disorders are elevated in gambling disorders, ongoing screening for problematic use of drugs and alcohol is highly encouraged. Clinicians are encouraged to use a Screening, Brief Intervention, and Referral to Treatment (SBIRT) approach with gambling disorder patients in order to comprehensively identify all patterns of problematic use. Switching addictions can occur during the course of recovery, further highlighting the need for clinicians to stay mindful of any signs of emerging addictions.

Suicidal ideation and suicide attempts are particularly elevated in gambling disorder and can occur at any time during the course of illness. Nearly 25% of all gambling disorder patients reported ongoing suicidality during the course of their condition. As a result, clinicians must be vigilant about screening and inquiring about the presence of self-injurious thoughts and then develop self-harm prevention plans. Elevated rates of suicidal ideation are thought to be due to the higher rates of impulsivity and risk taking seen in gamblers, as well as the desperation and hopelessness that can accompany staggering financial losses and problems.

Special Issues With Medical Comorbidities

Gambling disorder can affect physical health in a variety of ways: it primarily adversely affects quality of sleep and general self-care (diet and exercise) and raises the risk of stress-related health problems such as heart disease and hypertension. Gamblers have shown a higher use of the health care system and report lower overall quality of health as compared with nongamblers.

Epidemiological surveys have identified that having a medical disability of any kind increases a person's risk of developing a gambling disorder (Morasco and Petry 2006). This finding serves as a constant reminder to all clinicians to screen for gambling activity, no matter how physically or mentally disabled a patient may be. Unlike other forms of addiction that require in-person transactions and pursuits to acquire addictive substances, the satisfaction of gambling urges can be conducted in the comforts of home, as long as a person has access to credit and means with which to gamble.

Patients who have Parkinson's disease or restless legs syndrome or who currently take dopamine agonists should be cautioned about the possible emergence of gambling disorder, because of a documented association between dopamine agonists and gambling disorder. This side effect, although relatively rare, will manifest relatively quickly after initiation or dose escalation. Patients describe an insatiable urge to gamble, an absence of fear of losing money, and a loss of tension associated with risk-taking behaviors. In most cases, cessation of the dopamine agonist results in abatement of gambling disorder.

Special Issues With Specific Populations

Gambling disorder can develop across the life span, but adolescents and geriatric populations are particularly vulnerable and susceptible to not only developing a gambling disorder but also enduring the consequences of it.

ADOLESCENTS

Most casinos require patrons to be older than 21 to gamble, but adolescents have very easy access to gambling via nonregulated gambling activities in homes, in schools, and online, as well as underage gambling in legal venues. Adolescents who develop gambling disorders have been shown to be more likely to have co-occurring psychiatric problems and develop gambling disorders more quickly than do their adult counterparts. Gambling disorder in adolescents can manifest easily as declining academic performance, changes in personality, defiance, and any symptoms that mimic mood, anxiety, or ADHD conditions.

ELDERLY

The proliferation of gambling in the United States has reached the elderly population with ease. Casino buses, also called "turnarounds," offer cheap tickets to transport gamblers to and from local destinations. Nationally, the prevalence rate of gambling disorder among elderly persons is lower than in adult populations, but the clinical impact is much more intense and emotionally draining. Elderly gamblers who accrue large debts do so with profound effect on their families, at times creating generational debt and financial problems that cannot be resolved while on fixed incomes. The guilt, shame, and trauma of losing financial savings that took years to build can be a massive psychological trauma unlike in any other addictive disorders.

FEMALE GENDER

Recent treatment data and epidemiological data show that nearly 40% of all gambling disorder patients are female (Hing et al. 2015). This is a much higher percentage than in the 1970s and 1980s, which suggested a closing of the gender gap. Researchers have indicated that this change is a result of increasing acceptability of gambling among females, as well as improved problem gambling education initiatives that lead to treatment seeking. Traditionally, female gamblers have been stereotyped as slot machine players, but this stereotype no longer holds true because many female patients with gambling disorder play poker and casino table games.

What to Do About Other Behavioral Addictions

In addition to gambling disorder, the most common forms of behavioral addiction that patients present with in the clinical setting are hypersexual disorder, compulsive spending or shopping, Internet use disorder, and online gaming addiction. Scientifically accepted criteria have not been established for these other forms of behavioral addiction, but clinicians are encouraged to screen for and inquire about these behaviors because they do occur commonly.

Treatment plans for behavioral addiction are similar to treatment plans recommended for other addictive disorders—a biopsychosocial treatment approach with an integrated and multidisciplinary plan for recovery. At this time, no FDA-approved medications are available, and the evidence base for effective psychotherapies is very small. Clinicians borrow principles and treatment techniques from management of other addictive disorders and apply them to these conditions. Twelve-step groups (even some online) are available and can be used for support, community, and fellowship.

KEY POINTS

Gambling disorder is as prevalent in the general population as schizophrenia or bipolar disorder.

Screening for signs and symptoms of gambling disorder should occur at intake, at regular intervals, and especially with patients who have risk factors to develop gambling disorder.

Treatment for gambling disorder requires a biopsychosocial approach that uses an integrated, multidisciplinary team for recovery.

References

Achab S, Khazaal Y: Psychopharmacological treatment in pathological gambling: a critical review. Curr Pharm Des 17(14):1389–1395, 2011 21524264

American Psychiatric Association: Diagnostic and Statistical Manual of Mental Disorders, 3rd Edition. Washington, DC, American Psychiatric Association, 1980

American Psychiatric Association: Diagnostic and Statistical Manual of Mental Disorders, 4th Edition. Washington, DC, American Psychiatric Association, 1994

American Psychiatric Association: Diagnostic and Statistical Manual of Mental Disorders, 5th Edition. Arlington, VA, American Psychiatric Association, 2013

Gebauer L, LaBrie R, Shaffer HJ: Optimizing DSM-IV-TR classification accuracy: a brief biosocial screen for detecting current gambling disorders among gamblers in the general household population. Can J Psychiatry 55(2):82–90, 2010 20181303

Grant JE, Potenza MN, Weinstein A, et al: Introduction to behavioral addictions. Am J Drug Alcohol Abuse 36(5):233–241, 2010 20560821

Hing N, Russell A, Tolchard B, Nower L: Risk factors for gambling problems: an analysis by gender. J Gambl Stud 2015 May 7. [Epub ahead of print] 25948418

Hodgins DC, Stea JN, Grant JE: Gambling disorders. Lancet 378(9806):1874–1884, 2011 21600645

Johnson EE, Hammer R, Nora RM, et al: The Lie/Bet Questionnaire for screening pathological gamblers. Psychol Rep 80(1):83–88, 1997 9122356

Morasco BJ, Petry NM: Gambling problems and health functioning in individuals receiving disability. Disabil Rehabil 28(10):619–623, 2006 16690574

PART III

Treatment

CHAPTER 15

Cognitive-Behavioral Therapy

ADAM R. DEMNER, M.D.

COGNITIVE-behavioral therapy (CBT) is a short-term, problem-focused psychotherapy founded on the principles of behavioral learning theory. Developed by Aaron T. Beck, M.D., CBT is based on his cognitive model that dysfunctional thinking is common to all psychological disturbances; when this thinking is modified through careful and guided evaluation in a more adaptive way, individuals benefit from resolution of such disturbances.

The term "cognitive-behavioral therapy" has at times been used to describe *cognitive-behavioral treatments*, which can be thought of as an umbrella term that includes CBT with other therapeutic interventions such as relapse prevention and motivational interviewing. However, in this chapter, I focus on the principles and implementation of CBT as it relates to the key components of Beck's theory and psychotherapy, with particular emphasis on the conceptualization and treatment of substance use disorders.

Foundations of Cognitive-Behavioral Theory

This treatment was originally termed *cognitive therapy* by Beck, but it has become synonymous with the term *CBT* and was devised as a structured, problem-focused, short-term psychotherapy with the emphasis on dysfunctional behaviors, thoughts, and beliefs. In the treatment of substance use disorders, particular focus is placed on

- Negative beliefs about the self
- Permission-granting beliefs about substance use

For example, if negative beliefs about the self ("I don't deserve to feel good" or "I can't do it on my own") are heightened and permission-granting beliefs ("It's okay to have a drink; it's been a rough day" or "I can take just a few pills this time because nobody will ever know") become rampant, then the likelihood of ongoing use is high. Alternatively, if the self is viewed in a positive way and permission-granting beliefs are mitigated, then the individual has a higher likelihood of achieving and maintaining goals. Transforming these maladaptive cognitive dysfunctions into adaptive reality-based beliefs is at the core of CBT.

The cognitive-behavioral model is based on the hypothesis that people's perception of events can influence their emotions and behaviors but also considers the two primary types of learning:

1. Learning by association (classical conditioning)
2. Learning by consequences (operant conditioning)

Classical conditioning, or learning by association, is a process of behavioral learning in which a previously neutral stimulus triggers a strong biological reaction when paired repeatedly with a known biological reward. Such learning was made famous by Ivan Pavlov and his experiments conducted with dogs, who began to salivate at the sound of keys (previously neutral stimulus) that immediately preceded feeding time (known biological reward); thus, a biological reaction of salivation was reproduced by the sound of keys, a previously neutral stimulus. Classical conditioning is the basis for a cognitive conceptualization of triggers (i.e., people, places, and things) regarding the treatment of substance use disorders as well as the technique of functional analysis, described later in this chapter (see the section "Functional Analysis and Daily Thought Records").

Operant conditioning, or learning by consequences, is a method of learning that occurs through punishment or rewards for behavior and was popularized by B.F. Skinner, Ph.D. In this method of learning, behaviors can be either reinforced/enhanced by reward leading to repeated expression or eliminated/reduced if followed by punishment. For example, an individual addicted to crack cocaine may continue using despite the consequences or punishment (e.g., financial burden or risk of incarceration) if the benefits or rewards of use (euphoria or escape from negative feelings) are viewed by the individual as having more value. Principles of operant conditioning are the basis for "advantages-disadvantages analysis" (Beck et al. 1993), a technique of carefully weighing the potential rewards or punishments of ongoing substance use when applying CBT to the treatment of substance use disorders.

Basics of Cognitive-Behavioral Therapy

CBT is offered in a variety of settings (i.e., individual or groups) either as monotherapy or in conjunction with other treatments, ranging from motivational interviewing to 12-step facilitation to pharmacotherapy. Myriad specific therapies derived from Beck's original theories are beyond the scope of this chapter. However, the core principles are generally universal and can be outlined by the 10 principles in Table 15–1.

Structure of the Cognitive-Behavioral Therapy Session

The primary goal of the evaluation session is to establish an accurate diagnosis. Additional tasks include

- Formulating a cognitive conceptualization
- Determining whether additional treatments (e.g., medications) are indicated
- Initiating the therapeutic alliance
- Setting broad goals for treatment

It is important to clarify expectations early in the course of treatment and to allow for time to discuss termination as the treatment nears the end; after all, CBT aims to be a time-limited treatment.

Each subsequent session follows a similar general format, but rigidly following a script and ignoring the patient's lead may lead to difficulties; however, leaving the structure too loose will create its own difficulties. The skilled therapist will find the right balance between structure and flexibility depending on the patient's lead but will not stray too far from the problem-focused approach of CBT.

Sessions tend to begin by checking in on the identified goal of treatment followed by setting the agenda and clearly defin-

TABLE 15–1. Core principles of cognitive-behavioral therapy

1. Is based on an evolving conceptualization in cognitive terms
2. Necessitates a strong therapeutic alliance
3. Emphasizes collaborations and active participation
4. Is a problem-focused therapy
5. Emphasizes the here and now
6. Teaches patients to be their own therapist
7. Aims to be time-limited
8. Has structured sessions
9. Teaches patients to address their dysfunctional thoughts beyond the confines of the therapy session
10. Implements a variety of techniques to change cognitions, mood, and behavior

Source. Adapted from Beck 2011.

ing the goals for the current session. The therapist may say something to the effect of "Hello, Joe. How has your anxiety been this past week? Any specific issues that you have on your mind for today's session? If not, that's okay, I just wanted to be able to carve out some time for specific things if needed. If not, then let us see how you did with your homework."

If the patient has nothing specific on the agenda, the therapist can move to reviewing of homework or, as some patients prefer, assignments. Homework is an integral component of CBT and can take many forms:

- Behavioral activation (engaging in a specific behavior)
- Monitoring and evaluating automatic thoughts (as in the daily thought record, described later in this chapter; see the section "Functional Analysis and Daily Thought Records")
- Behavioral experiments (so patients can test the validity of their thoughts and beliefs)
- Bibliotherapy (having patients read about various concepts that arise in session)

If patients did not complete their homework, it might be helpful to explore why; for example, maybe Joe was too anxious to complete his homework and could benefit from more guidance in the session.

Figure 15–1 (adapted from Beck 2011) summarizes the key components of the cognitive model. This model is pivotal to the cognitive conceptualization, which is an evolving process that begins at the initial therapy session and is refined throughout treatment. This model hypothesizes that an individual's perceptions of a situation, which manifest as an automatic thought, can directly influence behavior. In other words, it is not necessarily the situation or trigger in and of itself but rather the way in which the situation is perceived that results in different reactions. However, vulnerable situations certainly warrant thorough exploration and understanding along with the perceptions thereof. These automatic thoughts are influenced by, and can be a window into, an individual's underlying system of beliefs. Such beliefs are influenced by early life experiences and current life problems.

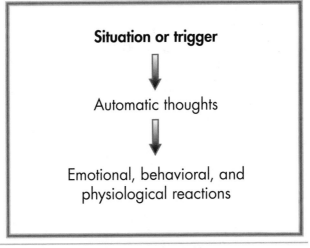

FIGURE 15–1.   Cognitive conceptualization.
Source.   Adapted from Beck 2011.

FUNCTIONAL ANALYSIS AND
DAILY THOUGHT RECORDS

Functional analysis, based on the principles of classical conditioning, is the identification of antecedents of and triggers for certain behaviors; when functional analysis is applied to the treatment of substance use disorders, the identified behavior is substance use. Individuals are more likely to be aware of an emotion or a behavior than they are of the automatic thought or the precipitating event. For example, an individual attempting to quit smoking may find himself or herself holding a lit cigarette without being fully cognizant of the emotional reaction, automatic thought, or triggering event.

Daily thought records can be used to expand functional analysis beyond the confines of the therapy session. In fact, assigning homework is an integral, not optional, technique of CBT. The core components of a thought record include

1. Detailed situation
2. Automatic thoughts
3. Accompanying emotions
4. Responses
5. Outcome

Applying this technique to the example above, the situation may have been as follows: 1) The aroma of tobacco smoke from a stranger nearby led to 2) the thought of "I really want a cigarette right now," 3) accompanied by an emotion of anxiety and a physiological response of craving, which influenced 4) a behavioral response of requesting a cigarette from a stranger; 5) the outcome was to relapse.

As treatment progresses, one of the goals is to develop more adaptive responses by evaluating the dysfunctional automatic thought *before* engaging in the behavior.

AUTOMATIC THOUGHTS

Once functional analysis and the daily thought record have been implemented, a maladaptive automatic thought will be identified. Automatic thoughts emerge from core beliefs and parallel a more noticeable stream of thought. Automatic thoughts are not necessarily pathological and are common to all, such as an individual who automatically thinks "I'm such an idiot" once realizing he forgot his wallet at home. These thoughts often occur without much notice and are best elicited from an active, collaborative, and nonjudgmental stance using open-ended questioning.

It is rarely beneficial to directly challenge a dysfunctional automatic thought, and Socratic questioning is a better approach. By understanding the identified thought in detail, the therapist can help the patient modify his or her thoughts, leading to alternative behavioral and emotional reactions. See Table 15–2 for some suggested questions regarding automatic thoughts, followed by an example dialogue (adapted from Beck 2011).

TABLE 15–2. Questions regarding automatic thoughts

1. What is the evidence for and against the thought?

2. Is there an alternative way to look at the situation?

3. What is the worst- and best-case scenario, the most realistic, and if it happened, could you cope?

4. What happens when you believe this thought to be true, and what might happen if your thinking were to change?

5. What would you tell _____ [family member or friend] if this was his or her situation?

6. What should you do?

THERAPIST (TH): Okay, Joe, so when you saw your friends doing cocaine, you thought, "I can control myself this time, and I need it to have fun with them." Is that right?

PATIENT (PT): Yeah.

TH: Well, let's take a look at this automatic thought. Is there any evidence that supports or goes against it?

PT: There was once a time when I could do just one or two lines, but that was a long time ago, and for the most part, I find myself losing control and then regretting it the next day.

TH: Seems that the evidence is not really in support of your idea that you can control your use. I wonder if there is another way of looking at this situation.

PT: It makes me think that maybe these aren't the *friends* I thought they were. I know I can't really have *just a little* of anything.

Cognitive-Behavioral Therapy

TH: That's an interesting point about the people you were associating with. What is the best-case scenario if this thought of being able to control yourself and needing cocaine to have fun were true?

PT: Well, I'd be able to go out, control myself, and have a good time. But it never really happens that way.

TH: OK, I'm hearing you. What is the worst-case outcome if this thought of controlling yourself and needing cocaine to have fun were true? And what do you think the most realistic outcome would be?

PT: The worst-case scenario is probably the most realistic. I'd probably lose control, end up having a terrible time, embarrassing myself, and feeling depressed the next day.

TH: Ahh, so when you believe this thought to be true, you ultimately lose control and end up embarrassed. What might happen if your thinking were to change? I'm not saying it would be easy, but if it were to happen?

PT: If I thought "Don't even touch that stuff; you know you'll lose control" and "Why are these *friends* doing coke in front of me?," I'd probably leave the situation and end up having fun with my other friends who don't use.

TH: Sounds like you're coming up with quite a few options. What do you think you would say to Zach, your friend who has been in recovery for a few years, if he was in the same situation?

PT: I'd tell him that he was crazy to think that he could actually have just one line. And I've known him for a year now—every time we hang out, we have a good time, and we never used any cocaine!

TH: So, any thoughts about what you might do if this situation comes up again?

PT: It seems so obvious now, but I guess I didn't even realize my automatic thought in the first place. Now I'll be more aware, realize that I have to get out of there, away from my *friends,* and I'll probably give Zach a call. I can have fun without coke—and come to think of it, most of the time I use, I end up having a bad time anyway.

INTERMEDIATE AND CORE BELIEFS

Automatic thoughts not only are a target for direct therapeutic intervention but also serve as a window into the patient's underlying beliefs; these beliefs can be divided into intermediate and core beliefs.

Intermediate beliefs are assumptions that serve the purpose of coping with core beliefs. These intermediate beliefs can be thought of as rules the individual lives by in order to tolerate negative core beliefs; each intermediate belief has a positive or negative counterpart. For example, someone who has the intermediate belief "If I am not in control, then something bad will happen" holds the positive belief "If I am always in control, then I will be safe."

Core beliefs are the most central idea that an individual has about his or her self. These can be categorized into three realms: 1) the helpless realm, 2) the unlovability realm, 3) and the worthlessness realm (Beck 2011). Core beliefs are unlikely to be manifested by these exact words, and the therapist should listen carefully for variants. Examples for the core belief "I am helpless" might come out as "I am broken," "I am out of control," "I am inferior," and "I am incapable." For the belief "I am unlovable," examples of what the patient may say include "I am not fun," "I am ugly," and "I am undesirable."

Identifying these beliefs can be more challenging than questioning automatic thoughts but takes a similar approach with Socratic questioning. The downward arrow technique (Burns 1980) begins with identification of a salient automatic thought that comes from a dysfunctional belief. By exploring the meaning of the automatic thought, the therapist can uncover important beliefs. Asking what a thought might mean *to* the patient can elicit an intermediate belief, whereas asking what the thought means *about* the patient might yield a core belief. Continuing with the earlier example of Joe's automatic thought will illustrate this technique:

TH: Good work questioning that automatic thought, Joe. Now that we have a better understanding of how it influences your behavior, I am curious as to what that specific thought means to you.

PT: The thought that I can control myself and that I need to be high on cocaine to have fun? I never really thought about it.

TH: Well, assume the thought is true for the moment. What does it mean for you to be in control of yourself?

PT: Hmmm, the first thing that comes to mind is that if I am in control, then I'll know exactly what to expect—I'll feel safe. But if I lose control, that's when bad things can happen.

TH: And what does that say about you? To lose control.

PT: I wouldn't be safe. I would be helpless.

TH: Any thoughts about thinking you need cocaine to have fun? What does it mean to you to need a drug to have fun?

PT: If I am high, then I will have a good time. On the flip
   side, if I am not high, then I won't have as much fun.
TH: Okay, I hear what you're saying. But what does that say
   about you as a person, that you think you won't have
   fun unless you are high?
PT: I don't know exactly what you mean. I have always
   been the life of the party; everybody knows who I am.
   I need to be fun—if I am not fun, then people won't
   like me.
TH: I see. And why do you need a substance to make you
   fun?
PT: I guess I don't feel good enough, like I'm broken or
   something. That nobody actually loves me.

ADDICTIVE BELIEFS

Beck et al. (1993) considers addictive beliefs in terms of ideas
related to seeking pleasure, solving problems, providing relief, and offering escape. Some of the various dysfunctional
addictive beliefs include

- A substance is necessary to maintain emotional and/or
  physical balance.
- The substance will improve functioning.
- The use of a substance will provide pleasure (supported
  by the belief that urges will worsen unless acted on).
- The substance is needed to relieve distress or escape from
  boredom.

In addition to these beliefs and ideas, there are permission-giving beliefs (Beck et al. 1993) relating to justification,
risk taking, and entitlement. Examples include

- "It's okay to have a drink; it's been a really hard day."
- "The relief I will get is worth the risk of slipping into a
  full-blown relapse."
- "I deserve some relief, and I'm entitled to have a drink if
  everyone else can."

COGNITIVE DISTORTIONS

The downward arrow technique can be a good tool to explore
dysfunctional thoughts and the underlying beliefs that support them. Another approach to evaluating these thoughts and
beliefs is with the use of *cognitive distortions,* also known as

thinking errors. It can be beneficial to label distortions collaboratively during the session and then model the technique so that the patient can implement it independently. The following list includes some common cognitive distortions, with examples relating to the treatment of substance use disorders:

- *All-or-nothing thinking:* Polarizing a situation rather than entertaining a spectrum of possibilities. Example: "If I slip and have one drink, I might as well go ahead and have another 15."
- *Catastrophizing:* Negatively predicting future events without clear reason to do so. Example: "I will have the worst time in my life unless I am high at that party."
- *Emotional reasoning:* Something is believed to be true because of intense feelings, notwithstanding a paucity of evidence. Example: "I know that I have so many months clean, but I still feel like I am a failure."
- *Minimization:* Ascribing insignificance to a seemingly important event. Example: "It isn't that bad; at least I didn't inject the heroin this time."
- *Selective abstraction:* Paying significant attention to one negative detail rather than the entire situation. Example: "I had one slip in 5 years; there is no way I can show up at a meeting now that I have failed."

CURRENT LIFE PROBLEMS AND RELEVANT CHILDHOOD DATA

In a similar manner that underlying beliefs influence automatic thoughts, additional factors influence these beliefs; such factors include current stressors and more remote childhood experiences. Current life problems include all the difficulties that an individual is experiencing beyond the scope of the identified problematic behavior. These include

- Academic or occupational difficulties
- Problems meeting basic needs of shelter or food
- Stressful interpersonal relationships
- Medical problems
- Legal issues

It can be helpful, albeit challenging, for the therapist to differentiate problems that lead to substance use from sequelae of use—sometimes the stressor can be both a cause and an effect of substance use, such as financial hardship.

Information from the patient's childhood, notwithstanding CBT's focus on the here and now, can be helpful to better understand how core beliefs came to be and how they might be perpetuated. For the treatment of substance use disorders, such information about early life experiences also can facilitate the understanding and modification of the patient's addictive beliefs. Consider the aforementioned example of Joe, who thinks that he can control his cocaine use and needs it to have (and be) fun, assumes he needs to have control to feel safe, and at the core believes that he is helpless and unlovable. Knowing that Joe was raised in a chaotic environment by substance-using parents may help to explain his feelings about control and safety. Additionally, understanding that his parents were neglectful in the context of *their* substance use may shed light on his core belief of being unlovable. Addictive beliefs were also likely influenced by the environment in which he was raised and may explain his permission-giving beliefs.

Evidence for Cognitive-Behavioral Therapy for Substance Use Disorders

Meta-analytic reviews of psychosocial interventions for substance use disorders and additional reviews have investigated the effect of cognitive-behavioral treatments; however, many of these publications broadly define "cognitive-behavioral therapy" to include a variety of treatments that differ from standard CBT as described in this chapter. Such treatments include motivational interviewing (see Chapter 17).

The COMBINE study was a randomized controlled trial evaluating the efficacy of medication, behavioral therapies, and their combinations in the treatment of alcohol dependence; in addition, the efficacy of combined behavioral intervention was studied. *Combined behavioral intervention* was defined as integrating aspects of CBT, 12-step facilitation, motivational interviewing, and an additional support system. The conclusions were that patients who received medical management with naltrexone (an opioid antagonist used to treat alcohol use disorder), combined behavioral intervention, or both had better drinking outcomes; however, the combination of naltrexone and combined behavioral intervention did not have an additive effect (Anton et al. 2006).

Notwithstanding the limitations, many of which are ubiquitous in psychotherapy research, evidence from numerous large-scale trials and reviews supports the efficacy of CBT for alcohol use disorders and other substance use disorders. One meta-analytic review of CBT for drug abuse and dependence included 34 randomized controlled trials and found an overall moderate effect size with larger effect sizes found for treatment of cannabis, followed by treatments of cocaine and opioids, and the smallest effect size for treatments of polysubstance dependence (McHugh et al. 2010).

KEY POINTS

Cognitive-behavioral therapy for substance use disorders is a problem-focused, time-limited, and evidence-based psychotherapeutic intervention aimed to uncover and restructure maladaptive automatic thoughts through a variety of individualized techniques.

Conceptualized from the cognitive-behavioral model, substance use disorders are viewed as learned behaviors (via classical and/or operant conditioning), precipitated and perpetuated by dysfunctional automatic thoughts and beliefs that are influenced by early life experiences and current life stressors.

Cognitive-behavioral therapy can be effectively used in conjunction with other treatment modalities, including pharmacotherapy, or integrated with techniques of relapse prevention and motivational interviewing.

References

Anton RF, O'Malley SS, Ciraulo DA, et al: Combined pharmacotherapies and behavioral interventions for alcohol dependence: the COMBINE study: a randomized controlled trial. JAMA 295(17): 2003–2017, 2006 16670409

Beck AT, Wright FD, Newman CF, et al: Cognitive Therapy of Substance Abuse. New York, Guilford, 1993

Beck J: Cognitive Behavior Therapy: Basics and Beyond, 2nd Edition. New York, Guilford, 2011

CHAPTER 16

Relapse Prevention

BERNADINE HAN, M.D., M.S.

JONATHAN AVERY, M.D.

RELAPSE prevention is an approach to the treatment of substance use disorders originally developed for alcohol use disorder by Alan Marlatt and his colleagues in the 1970s. The effectiveness and efficacy of relapse prevention have been shown repeatedly for multiple substance use disorders, including alcohol, nicotine, cocaine, and opioids, with the most consistent evidence seen in the treatment of alcohol use disorders. Relapse prevention has been shown to work in both outpatient and inpatient settings and may be most helpful for individuals with high levels of impairment (in terms of both substance use and psychopathology). Relapse prevention does not always prevent relapse, but it can significantly decrease the negative consequences that may result after returning to substance use. Unlike most other treatments that have fading effects over time, relapse prevention also has demonstrated a "delayed emergence effect." This effect has been attributed to the development of new coping skills that individuals build when encountering lapses; these skills prevent future relapse.

Models of Relapse

LAPSE, RELAPSE, RECOVERY

Although relapse is often considered an end point per se, in terms of relapse prevention, it is probably more helpful to understand relapse as a process. As defined by Marlatt and Gordon (1985):

- A *lapse* is the first time an individual uses a substance after a period of abstinence. Lapses are very likely to happen in the process of trying to change a behavior.
- A *relapse* occurs when an individual continues to use a substance after an initial lapse. The pattern of relapse use may mirror previous problematic substance use.
- *Prolapse (recovery)* is behavior that is consistent with desired behavior change, whether the goal is abstinence or more moderate use.

Other definitions of relapse are common; some use numerical cutoffs (e.g., days of use), whereas others try to incorporate the effect that the return to substance use may have on the individual's life and functioning.

COGNITIVE-BEHAVIORAL MODEL

Relapse prevention often makes use of a cognitive-behavioral model, with a particular focus on what is known as the *abstinence violation effect* (AVE). The AVE refers to the guilt and blame that a person feels after breaking self-imposed rules. This frequently leads to feelings of futility, lost effort, and failure that can facilitate the transition from lapse to relapse. The AVE comprises both

- An affective component
- A cognitive component

The affective side is triggered by the conflict inherent in having used a substance while the individual has begun to believe in himself or herself as an abstainer. The cognitive framing of the events leading up to the lapse is also an important part of the AVE. The ability to see the contributing factors as controllable and modifiable, as opposed to inevitable and unavoidable, can protect an individual from believing that lapse represents failure—a belief that can turn lapse to relapse. Instead, the individual may be more likely to accept the occasion as an opportunity to examine the circumstances leading up to the lapse and to develop more effective coping skills to prevent similar lapses in the future.

Because of its importance in the transition from lapse to relapse, the AVE is an important target of the cognitive-behavioral model of relapse, which hinges on how an individual responds to a high-risk situation. The cognitive-behavioral model describes relapse as a linear process, grounded in a matrix of environmental or interpersonal and personal risk factors (Figure 16–1). External cues create a trigger to use substances, internal coping resources shape the individual's response to that trigger, and the ultimate decision to use weighs an individual's coping skills against the anticipated outcome of use.

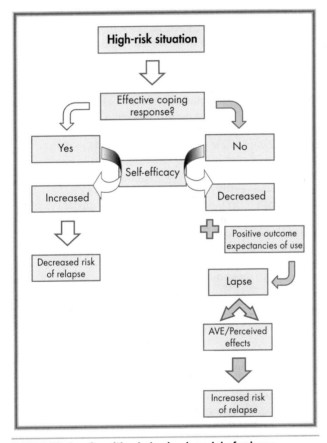

FIGURE 16–1. Cognitive-behavioral model of relapse.

A linear progression toward relapse hinges on the individual's ability to cope in a high-risk situation. AVE=abstinence violation effect.

Source. Adapted from Marlatt and Gordon 1985.

DYNAMIC MODEL

The Relapse Replication and Extension Project, spearheaded by the National Institute on Alcohol Abuse and Alcoholism in 1996, investigated Marlatt's original cognitive-behavioral model of relapse. As summarized by Douaihy et al. (2014), the conclusions corroborated the original findings that negative emotional states and social pressure created the most common high-risk situations for relapse, but otherwise found that the predictive ability of the original model was limited. These findings led to the development and proposal of a new model of relapse to account for the reality that the relapse process is not linear but rather random, complex, and fluid.

The dynamic model of relapse was proposed by Marlatt and Witkiewitz (2005) to account for the way that some risk factors and protective mechanisms remain constant over time but others vary by situation or context. Distal risks (such as years of use and family history) remain stable, whereas proximal risks, including a bad mood or passing by a liquor store, are immediate and triggering. Cognitive, behavioral, affective, and physical processes all play a role in the development of a high-risk scenario (Figure 16–2). This model allows for the reality that a small change may have a large downstream effect, depending on the circumstances of the moment in time and space. The model allows an individual to imagine and identify the ways in which different processes can come together to create a high-risk situation, which can facilitate a focused attempt at creating contingencies and coping skills for these different possibilities.

Basic Principles of Relapse Prevention

Relapse prevention treatment begins with the initial assessment of potential high-risk relapse situations, which may include factors of personality, social interaction, environment, and physiology. Cognitive and behavioral approaches at intervention and management are then applied to these identified triggers and situations. Part of this process involves cognitive restructuring of maladaptive thoughts and positive outcome expectancies. Lapse management, which specifically targets the AVE, is also an important cognitive intervention that can keep patients from seeing a lapse as a failure and help them understand relapse as a process.

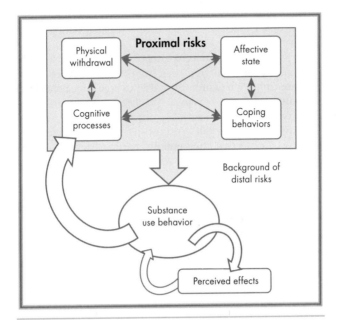

FIGURE 16–2. **Dynamic model of relapse.**
On a background of stable distal risks, more variable proximal risks interact with one another in dynamic ways to create potential high-risk situations for use, which affect future proximal risk.
Source. Adapted from Witkiewitz and Marlatt 2004.

DETERMINANTS OF LAPSE AND RELAPSE

Determinants of lapse and relapse are typically divided into the intrapersonal and interpersonal determinants.

INTRAPERSONAL DETERMINANTS

Intrapersonal determinants include the following:

- *Self-efficacy* describes how confident an individual may be in his or her ability to respond to a situation in a desired way. Self-efficacy is difficult to assess and quantify, but low self-efficacy is predictive of relapse.
- *Outcome expectancies* are the effects an individual expects (or hopes for) by using a substance (or indulging in other addictive behavior). These may be positive (e.g., better mood, easier social interactions) or negative. The expecta-

tion may not match the actual effects, and in fact the reality may be the opposite of what was anticipated. Negative outcome expectancies tend to be associated with positive treatment outcomes.

- *Craving* is the cognitive experience of wanting to use a substance. (This is differentiated from an *urge,* defined as the actual intention or impulse to use; an urge is the behavioral manifestation of craving.) Craving is, not surprisingly, strongly related to positive outcome expectancies, but craving itself has not been consistently predictive of relapse. Adjunctive interventions, particularly medications and mindfulness or meditation, can be useful in addressing craving.

- *Motivation* to change and motivation to use are the two relevant motivations in relapse prevention. The stages of change (precontemplation, contemplation, preparation, action, maintenance) are often used when assessing motivation to change and to increase ambivalence toward motivation to use. Motivation to change is specific; it may not include motivation for treatment, for example, or it may indicate motivation to stop using one substance while continuing to use another. Although high motivation to change is an important protective factor against relapse, it requires strong coping skills. Motivational interviewing addresses ambivalence toward change and conflicts between values and behaviors (for further discussion see Chapter 17, "Motivational Interviewing"). By doing this, motivational interviewing strengthens commitment to change and leads to better treatment outcomes.

- *Coping* is the most important predictor in the cognitive-behavioral model of relapse. *Approach coping* involves efforts to confront, accept, and reframe, whereas *avoidance coping* is based on distraction. Both methods appear to decrease relapse risk. Meditation techniques have been used in approach coping by facilitating the identification and acceptance of urges. "Urge surfing," cultivated through mindfulness, encourages an individual to observe urges without struggling with them.

- *Emotional states* have strong links to relapse. Outcome expectancies often target affect regulation—in some cases, substance use dulls or dissipates negative emotions or stress, but in others, it amplifies or reinforces an already positive affective state. Substance use can also relieve withdrawal states that may lead to negative affect.

INTERPERSONAL DETERMINANTS

Interpersonal determinants refer specifically to social supports. Social and emotional supports are strong predictors of long-term abstinence in various addictions, whereas interpersonal conflict and negative social pressure unsurprisingly increase risk of relapse. Behavioral marital therapy is an evidence-based approach to alcohol use disorder that incorporates partners in treatment.

RELAPSE PREVENTION STRATEGIES

Specific relapse prevention strategies in working with patients that aim to reduce lapse and the risk of relapse are listed here:

- Reconceptualize relapse as a process while improving the ability to identify its warning signs. Reviewing the connections among thoughts, feelings, events, situations, and using can bring insight to a patient's pattern of use.
- Identify high-risk situations and develop the cognitive and behavioral skills to cope with them. Understanding how each individual's high-risk situations are unique can maximize the benefit of skills training sessions, behavioral rehearsal, and cognitive reframing exercises.
- Develop communication skills and work on improving relationships with others. This tactic facilitates the development of a recovery social network. Pruning a patient's social network to exclude people who create pressure to use and rehearsing requests for support are important parts of this strategy.
- Learn how to identify negative emotional states and to manage and reduce their occurrence. The commonly used acronym HALT reminds patients not to let themselves become too **H**ungry, **A**ngry, **L**onely, or **T**ired.
- Build awareness of cravings and the cues that cause them. This can allow an individual to build or identify the tools to help manage them. Cue extinction techniques, avoidant coping, and mindfulness-based relapse prevention are all evidence-based approaches.
- Recognize and challenge cognitive distortions by pointing out patterns of unhelpful reasoning (generalizing, catastrophizing) and use-minimizing language.

Relapse Prevention　　　　　　　　　　　　　　**279**

- Work to develop a balanced lifestyle, with the goal of both reducing stress and building positive habits that can stand in for previous use behaviors.
- Consider adjunctive treatments, including medications and mindfulness-based practices, with psychosocial treatments.
- Facilitate transitions between levels of care when the patient is leaving residential or inpatient programs and again when the patient is leaving partial hospitalization or intensive outpatient programs. Even a single motivational therapy session before discharge and telephone or mail reminders of outpatient appointments have been shown to increase rates of treatment adherence after discharge.
- Work on ways to improve adherence to treatment and medications. Unsurprisingly, better adherence is associated with better outcomes.

Adjunct Treatments in Relapse Prevention

Adjunct treatments have been shown to improve outcomes in most substance-using populations and may be particularly useful among patients with comorbid psychiatric diagnoses.

MEDICATIONS

Adjunct medications are frequently used in the treatment of various substance use disorders and may help in preventing relapse as well. One explanation for this effect is that medications target physical and biological aspects of abstaining from substances that are ineffectively addressed by the behavioral and cognitive tools that relapse prevention develops. (The use of these medications is discussed more extensively in separate chapters.) For an alcohol use disorder, naltrexone, acamprosate, disulfiram, and a host of other medications have been shown to be effective. Nicotine replacement therapy, especially in combination with behavioral therapy, has consistently shown benefit when used for smoking cessation. Methadone, L-α-acetylmethadol, buprenorphine, naltrexone, and other medications have been used in opioid use disorder. Although some options may prove helpful in individual cases, no medications have consistently been found better than placebo when used in cocaine and cannabis use disorders.

MINDFULNESS AND MEDITATION

Mindfulness-based treatments incorporate the individual's development of nonjudgmental and nonreactive awareness to his or her emotional and physical states. This awareness can strengthen approach-based coping skills and thereby help individuals identify and use contingencies. Meditation and other mindfulness practices have been shown to decrease relapse (Bowen et al. 2014), with evidence of better long-term outcomes in reducing drug use and heavy drinking compared with relapse prevention alone. Meditation interventions also have been effectively used in depression, personality disorders, stress reduction, and irritable bowel syndrome.

Effectiveness of Relapse Prevention

The accumulation of data supporting the efficacy of relapse prevention in treating substance use disorder has led to the inclusion of relapse prevention in the U.S. Substance Abuse and Mental Health Services Administration's National Register of Evidence-Based Programs and Practices (Douaihy et al. 2014). A narrative review of randomized controlled trials of relapse prevention in the treatment of different substance use disorders (Carroll 1996) found that relapse prevention

- Was significantly better than no treatment
- Had mixed results compared with other therapeutic interventions
- Decreased the effect of relapse when it happened
- Increased the duration of positive treatment effects
- Proved particularly effective in patients with comorbid psychiatric illness, as well as in those whose substance use was correlated with worse affect, greater physical dependence on the substance, and other measures of impairment

In a separate meta-analysis (Irvin et al. 1999), relapse prevention was found to be effective in decreasing substance use. More markedly, treatment with relapse prevention was correlated with improvements in mood, coping skills, relationships, sense of agency, and other markers of psychosocial adjustment. The same study noted relapse prevention's efficacy with alcohol use disorder (most significantly), polysubstance use disorders, and smoking. It also found relapse prevention to be useful in both inpatient and outpatient settings and across individual, group, and marital therapies.

KEY POINTS

Although relapse has been known to be complex, dynamic, and unpredictable, disease models have tended to describe a linear path toward relapse. A new dynamic model of relapse has been proposed to better illustrate the multiple processes—internal and external, situational and constant—and the changing vulnerabilities that put an individual at risk for relapse.

The goals of relapse prevention are to prevent an initial lapse and, if a lapse occurs, to develop skills and techniques to help patients prevent or manage further relapse. This is done through an assessment and analysis of the intrapersonal and interpersonal factors that make a patient vulnerable to lapse, which allows for the identification of strategies to protect against those factors.

Evidence indicates that relapse prevention is most effective when used in alcohol use disorders. More research is warranted to improve outcomes in other substance use disorders, as well as to further refine the tools and techniques currently used to effect desired behavior change.

References

Bowen S, Witkiewitz K, Clifasefi SL, et al: Relative efficacy of mindfulness-based relapse prevention, standard relapse prevention, and treatment as usual for substance use disorders: a randomized clinical trial. JAMA Psychiatry 71(5):547–556, 2014 24647726

Carroll KM: Relapse prevention as a psychosocial treatment: a review of controlled clinical trials. Exp Clin Psychopharmacol 4(1):46–64, 1996

Douaihy A, Daley DC, Marlatt GA, et al: Relapse prevention: clinical models and intervention strategies, in The ASAM Principles of Addiction Medicine, 5th Edition. Edited by Ries RK, Fiellin DA, Miller SC, et al. Philadelphia, PA, Lippincott Williams & Wilkins, 2014, pp 991–1007

Irvin JE, Bowers CA, Dunn ME, et al: Efficacy of relapse prevention: a meta-analytic review. J Consult Clin Psychol 67(4):563–570, 1999 10450627

Marlatt GA, Gordon JR (eds): Relapse Prevention: Maintenance Strategies in the Treatment of Addictive Behaviors. New York, Guilford, 1985

Marlatt GA, Witkiewitz K: Relapse prevention for alcohol and drug problems, in Relapse Prevention: Maintenance Strategies in the Treatment of Addictive Behaviors, 2nd Edition. Edited by Marlatt GA, Donovan DM. New York, Guilford, 2005, pp 1–43

Witkiewitz K, Marlatt GA: Relapse prevention for alcohol and drug problems: that was Zen, this is Tao. Am Psychol 59(4):224–235, 2004 15149263

CHAPTER 17

Motivational Interviewing

JOHN DOUGLAS, M.D., M.B.A.

MOTIVATIONAL interviewing is a counseling approach that enhances the intrinsic motivation of people to change their behaviors. This technique was first described by William Miller, Ph.D., in his 1983 article, "Motivational Interviewing With Problem Drinkers," published in *Behavioural Psychiatry*. Over the years, he refined it in collaboration with Stephen Rollnick, Ph.D. Their book, *Motivational Interviewing: Helping People Change*, is the definitive work on the subject (Miller and Rollnick 2013). They define *motivational interviewing* for the layperson as "a collaborative conversation style for strengthening a person's own motivation and commitment to change" (p. 12). This counseling style is particularly effective for people addicted to substances but also can be used to help people make a variety of positive behavioral changes. Since the development of motivational interviewing, numerous clinical trials and meta-analyses have shown this approach to be effective in treating both addictive disorders and potentially related comorbid diseases, such as hypertension, HIV infection, diabetes, and obesity (Miller and Rollnick 2013). All of these conditions improve when patients change their behaviors.

Spirit

Motivational interviewing encompasses a variety of skills and strategies that often blend together. When using this counseling approach, it is helpful to keep in mind the spirit of motivational interviewing. The essence of the spirit is to see the best in people from their own unique perspectives and evoke from them the strengths they already possess to make behavioral changes. The spirit has four important interrelated elements, which are detailed in the following sections.

PARTNERSHIP

In motivational interviewing, practitioners and patients partner together. This partnership is very different from the typical relationship between practitioners and patients, in which it is common for practitioners to tell patients what to do. That strategy often generates resistance in the patient, which makes the interaction feel more like a struggle, somewhat akin to wrestling. In contrast, with motivational interviewing, the conversation between practitioners and patients should feel more like dancing, in which both participants move with each other rather than against each other.

ACCEPTANCE

Acceptance emphasizes valuing the absolute worth of patients as individuals and supporting their autonomy to make decisions for themselves. Practitioners communicate acceptance through expressing empathy, which conveys understanding from a patient's point of view. Acceptance is also communicated through affirming each patient's strengths and efforts. In general, patients feel accepted when they perceive that practitioners are searching to see what is "right" rather than what is "wrong" with them.

COMPASSION

Maintaining an attitude of compassion helps ensure that practitioners use motivational interviewing for the benefit of patients and not themselves. Motivational interviewing can be very effective and powerful, and if used without compassion, it could unfairly influence people. When it is exercised with compassion, practitioners pursue the best interests of patients.This ensures that the trust gained from patients is deserved and works for their benefit.

EVOCATION

Motivational interviewing assumes that patients already possess the strengths and resources they need to make personal changes in their lives. However, their awareness of these strengths and resources is often clouded by ambivalent feelings about making changes. The role of the practitioner in motivational interviewing is to evoke from patients an awareness of the strengths and resources they already possess and in the process to build their confidence to make personal changes. This is analogous to drawing water from a well. The implicit message from practitioners to patients is that they already have what they need, and together they will find it.

General Principles

Consistent with the spirit of motivational interviewing, the general principles of this counseling approach help guide responses to patients. These general principles can be easily remembered by the acronym REDS (Levounis and Arnaout 2010):

- *Roll with resistance:* Acknowledge the concerns of patients and avoid argumentative or confrontational statements. Confronting patients often puts them on the defensive and encourages them to justify their current behaviors, which prompts them to think of reasons not to change.
- *Express empathy:* Maintain a supportive and nonjudgmental attitude that conveys understanding from each patient's perspective. When patients feel understood, they often become more open to new ideas and ways of changing their behaviors.
- *Develop discrepancy:* Help patients identify areas where their current behaviors are inconsistent with achieving their goals. Recognizing these inconsistencies often instills in patients motivation to make behavioral changes more consistent with living the lives they want.
- *Support self-efficacy:* Highlight for patients their admirable qualities and past successes making behavioral changes, regardless of how minimal or short-lived they seem. Focusing on these positives helps build confidence for patients in making future behavioral changes.

Asking Permission

When topics come up with patients and they would benefit from making behavioral changes, be sure to ask for permission to explore these areas further. Asking permission communicates respect and lowers the resistance of patients, enabling the discussion of sensitive subjects such as substance use. Examples of asking permission include the following:

- "Do you mind if we talk about your smoking?"
- "You mentioned blacking out last week after drinking; do you mind if we talk about that further?"
- "I noticed from your previous records that you have a history of using cocaine. Do you mind if we talk about how that is going?"

Change Talk

Change talk is defined as statements by patients that favor movement in the direction of change. One of the main goals when using motivational interviewing is to enhance change talk from patients related to particular behaviors. In contrast, change talk differs from *sustain talk,* which is defined as statements by patients that indicate resistance to change. A higher ratio of change talk to sustain talk is associated with patients more successfully making behavioral changes.

The two main types of change talk to listen for are 1) preparatory change talk and 2) mobilizing change talk. Both types should be highlighted and encouraged from patients when using motivational interviewing.

PREPARATORY CHANGE TALK

Preparatory change talk is defined as statements from patients that indicate thoughts of how making changes would be better than continuing current behaviors. These statements signal the following and can be remembered by the acronym DARN:

Desire to change *(want, wish, hope)*

- "I want to quit smoking someday."
- "I wish I could drink like a normal person."
- "I hope to get better grades next year."

Ability to change *(can, could)*

- "I can have fun without alcohol."
- "I could go to rehab."

Reasons to change *(if…then)*

- "If I quit smoking at night, I would sleep better."
- "If I stopped spending my money on drugs, I could get an apartment."

Need to change *(need to, have to, must)*

- "I need to stop going out to bars every night."
- "I have to spend more time with my family."
- "I must get clean to keep my job."

MOBILIZING CHANGE TALK

Mobilizing change talk involves statements from patients that indicate a commitment to making changes now. These statements are even stronger than preparatory change talk and indicate current desires to make behavioral changes. They can be remembered by the acronym CAT:

Commitment *(intend, guarantee, promise)*

- "I intend to stop smoking marijuana every day."
- "I guarantee I will not use cocaine again."
- "I promise to be a better father to my children."

Activation *(willing, ready, prepared)*

- "I am willing to give up chewing tobacco."
- "I am ready to quit smoking."
- "I am prepared to eat healthier."

Taking steps *(went to, tried, started)*

- "I went to a support group meeting."
- "I tried not smoking any cigarettes yesterday."
- "I started looking into rehab programs."

Core Skills

Motivational interviewing uses four main skills to elicit change talk from patients. These skills can be remembered by the acronym OARS: 1) Open-ended questions, 2) Affirmations, 3) Reflections, and 4) Summaries.

OPEN-ENDED QUESTIONS

Open-ended questions cannot be answered in a single word. They should be used to initiate conversation and learn what is important to patients. Interspersing them with multiple reflections and affirmations helps patients feel heard and empowered, as in the following examples:

- "What brings you here today?"
- "How has this problem affected your day-to-day life?"
- "Where do you think this path that you're on is leading you?"
- "Is there anything you would like to change about your life?"
- "If you did decide to change, how would your life be different?"
- "What are the three best reasons for doing this?"

AFFIRMATIONS

Affirmations are statements that recognize and acknowledge strengths of patients. Using them increases the confidence of patients to successfully make changes. They often start with "you," as in the following examples:

- "You have made some big changes in the past."
- "You've thought a lot about this."
- "You have a lot to offer."

REFLECTIONS

Reflections can be simple or complex. Both types of reflections help patients to deepen their understanding of why making particular changes would be helpful. However, complex reflections are often more effective at eliciting change talk.

Simple reflections restate or rephrase what patients have already said. For example, if a patient says, "I'm feeling pretty depressed today," some potential simple reflections to this statement are as follows:

- "You're feeling depressed."
- "You're feeling kind of down."

Complex reflections offer interpretations of what patients say to expose their underlying meanings. The following are the main types of complex reflections:

- *Feeling:* "You are sad about this loss."
- *Metaphor:* "You see the light at the end of the tunnel."

- *Paraphrase and continue:* "It's been on your mind, and you're wondering what to do next."
- *Amplified:* "There is absolutely nothing you could do differently that would help."
- *Double-sided:* "The medication helps you feel better, but you don't want to become dependent on it."

SUMMARIES

When talking with patients, clinicians should summarize the change talk and present it back to them. This skill helps move patients forward in making changes. After giving a summary, it is helpful to ask, "What would you like to do next?" This question prompts patients to think about the initial steps of changing their behaviors.

Some patients may be unsure what to do next. For them, clinicians might try asking, "Would you like to hear suggestions of what other people have found helpful?" If the patient agrees, any relevant treatment strategies should be described. This approach is very different from standard interviewing, in which clinicians simply give advice without asking if patients want to hear it. Asking permission before sharing advice communicates respect and helps patients be more open to suggestions.

Evoking Change Talk

With use of the core skills of motivational interviewing, specific strategies have emerged that help evoke change talk. These strategies make change talk more likely to occur and are summarized in the following sections.

ASKING EVOCATIVE QUESTIONS

Evocative questions are open-ended questions for which change talk is the answer. The following are examples:

- "How would you like for things to change?"
- "What do you hope our work will accomplish?"
- "What don't you like about how things are now?"
- "How do you want your life to be different a year from now?"
- "If you did decide to get sober, how could you do it?"
- "What do you think you might be able to change?"

- "Of these various options you have considered, what seems most possible?"
- "Why would you want to stop smoking?"
- "You mentioned that your wife really gets on you about your drinking. If she were here now, what would she say are her concerns?"
- "What do you think has to change?"

USING A CHANGE RULER

A change ruler is an imaginary ruler ranging from 0 to 10 on which patients rate the importance to them of making specific behavioral changes. Asking the following three questions related to the change ruler encourages change talk and helps prompt patients to make changes:

1. First ask, "On a scale of 0 to 10, with 0 being not important at all and 10 being extremely important, how important is it to you right now to [insert behavior]?" This question also may be rephrased to assess the confidence of a patient in a plan to make a particular change, which is described further in the "Change Plan" section later in this chapter.
2. Then ask the follow-up question, "Why did you not say 0 [or lower number than the patient said]?" This question encourages change talk from the patient.
3. Finally ask, "What could happen to raise your answer to an 8 or 9 [or higher number than the patient said]?" This question builds on change talk from the previous question and encourages more.

QUERYING EXTREMES

Ask patients to describe extreme outcomes related to making a change or not. These outcomes may be positive or negative. Exploring the extremes of what may happen is particularly helpful when patients express little desire for change at present. Examples are as follows:

- "Suppose you continue on as you have been, without changing. What do you imagine are the worst things that could happen?"
- "What do you think could be the best results if you did make this change?"

LOOKING BACK

Ask patients to remember a time before a problematic behavior began, such as abusing substances, and compare that time with the present. The following are examples:

- "Do you remember a time when things were going well for you? What has changed?"
- "What were things like before you started using drugs? What were you like back then?"
- "What are the differences between the person you were 10 years ago and the person you are today?"

LOOKING FORWARD

Invite patients to think about what will likely happen in the future if they change their behaviors now and if they do not. This strategy is similar to querying extremes but more focused on what realistically will happen rather than the worst- or best-case scenarios. Examples are as follows:

- "If you decide to make this change, what would likely be different in the future?"
- "Suppose you don't make any changes but just continue as you have been. What do you think your life will be like in 5 years?"

EXPLORING GOALS AND VALUES

Discuss with patients their broader goals and values. This is helpful when used early in treatment sessions to develop rapport. It also helps patients identify what they value most and evaluate if their current behaviors will likely result in achieving their goals. Recognizing discrepancies between their current behaviors and stated goals or values evokes change talk. The following are some examples:

- "You seem like a person who values caring for your family. How does using drugs fit with that or not?"
- "How does [insert behavior] fit with what you want for your life?"

Change Plan

When a patient would like to make a behavioral change now or in the near future, clinicians should transition to developing a change plan. This is the specific plan the patient will follow to accomplish the change. Making a change plan may be appropriate after the first session but might not occur until after multiple sessions. Clinicians should keep in mind to always roll with resistance and not to push making a change plan if the patient is not ready. This is an essential concept in motivational interviewing. Pushing a patient toward change is often counterproductive and usually makes the patient less likely to change.

Change plans are usually most effective when focused on a specific behavioral change to make in the next 1 or 2 weeks. Developing these plans often varies from patient to patient. The following procedure highlights helpful questions to ask in the process:

- First ask, "What steps would you like to take in the next week or two to accomplish this change?"
- After the patient describes these steps, ask, "So that I'm clear, would you please summarize your plan?" Be sure that the patient gives the summary. This helps the patient solidify the plan.
- Then, use the change ruler with phrasing to assess the patient's confidence in the plan. Ask, "On a scale of 0 to 10, with 0 being not confident at all and 10 being extremely confident, how confident do you feel about carrying out this plan?" If the patient gives any number less than 7, inquire if anything can be changed about the plan to raise the patient's confidence to a higher number. Suggest a specific number that does not seem out of reach, such as 8 or 9. Explain that when confidence is 7 or more, people succeed more often in completing their plans. The patient may then choose to modify the plan or come up with a completely new one.
- Once the patient feels very confident about the change plan, do not raise any resistance, even if the plan has a low chance of success. Instead, affirm the patient and ask, "Would you like any follow-up with me to check in and see how the plan is going?" If the patient agrees, suggest how the patient can follow up with you.

- At the next session, ask, "How did it go with your plan?" Affirm any progress, regardless of how small. Then help the patient explore what worked and what did not. Continue to use motivational interviewing, and before ending the session, ask, "What would you like to do next?" Repeat this process at future sessions as long as the patient would like to continue working toward the desired behavioral change.

KEY POINTS

Motivational interviewing is a counseling approach that enhances the intrinsic motivation of people to change their behaviors.

The spirit of motivational interviewing is to see the best in people from their own unique perspectives and evoke from them the strengths they already possess to make behavioral changes.

The general principles of motivational interviewing emphasize using a supportive and nonconfrontational approach to help patients identify discrepancies between their current behaviors and future goals.

The central goal when using motivational interviewing is to enhance change talk, which is defined as statements by patients that favor making behavioral changes. Four core skills are used to elicit change talk and can be remembered by the acronym OARS: open-ended questions, affirmations, reflections, and summaries. Keep rowing with your OARS until you hear change talk.

To further evoke change talk, specific strategies based on the core skills of motivational interviewing are often helpful. These strategies include asking evocative questions, using the change ruler, querying extremes, looking back, looking forward, and exploring goals and values.

When patients would like to make changes now or in the near future, clinicians should transition to developing change plans, which are usually most successful when focused and specific.

References

Levounis P, Arnaout B: Handbook of Motivation and Change. Washington, DC, American Psychiatric Publishing, 2010

Miller WR: Motivational interviewing with problem drinkers. Behavioural Psychotherapy 11(2):147–172, 1983

Miller WR, Rollnick S: Motivational Interviewing: Helping People Change, 3rd Edition. New York, Guilford, 2013

CHAPTER 18

Twelve-Step Programs and Spirituality

J. DAVID STIFFLER, M.D.
EMILY DERINGER, M.D.

What Are 12-Step Programs?

Twelve-step programs encompass numerous organizations built on the principle of individuals working in fellowship to stop drinking, using other drugs, or other behaviors that are causing difficulty in their lives. The largest and most well-known 12-step program is Alcoholics Anonymous (AA). AA defines itself as

> an international fellowship of men and women who have had a drinking problem. It is nonprofessional, self-supporting, multiracial, apolitical, and available almost everywhere. There are no age or education requirements. Membership is open to anyone who wants to do something about his or her drinking problem. (Alcoholics Anonymous 2015)

The main principles of AA stem from both the historical roots in the founders' personal narratives and the belief in AA as a mechanism for change. These principles are articulated in the literature published by the organization—most notably, *Alcoholics Anonymous: The Story of How Many Thousands of Men and Women Have Recovered From Alcoholism* (Alcoholics Anonymous 2001), which is commonly referred to as *The Big Book*.

Twelve Steps

AA and other 12-step programs are rooted in a foundation of a 12-step progression (Table 18–1) through which members work, often with the encouraging aid of a sponsor. The *sponsor* is usually an individual of the same gender who has at least 1 year (often more) of sobriety. Some AA meetings focus on discussion of one of the steps (commonly referred to as *step meetings*), although often individuals will devote time outside the meetings, both individually and with their sponsor, to progress through the steps, more commonly referred to as *working the steps*.

AA also defines Twelve Traditions, which focus on the importance of the group and of anonymity. The Twelve Traditions explain that the "only requirement for AA membership is a desire to stop drinking" and describe that the AA groups are autonomous and self-supporting. Additionally, the Twelve Traditions state that AA

- Does not accept outside contributions
- Does not lend its name to any outside enterprises
- Does not take a position on outside issues

The Twelve Promises focus on what the alcoholic individual can try to attain by engaging in the program, emphasizing values such as happiness, peace, and loss of self-seeking and self-pity (Alcoholics Anonymous 2015).

Types of 12-Step Programs

AA is the oldest and largest of the 12-step programs and is the foundation on which many other 12-step programs are built. Narcotics Anonymous (NA) is the second largest of the 12-step groups and is open to anyone addicted to drugs, regardless of the type of drug. Other 12-step programs include

- Cocaine Anonymous
- Marijuana Anonymous
- Crystal Meth Anonymous
- Nicotine Anonymous

TABLE 18–1. Twelve Steps of Alcoholics Anonymous

1. We admitted we were powerless over alcohol—that our lives had become unmanageable.

2. Came to believe that a Power greater than ourselves could restore us to sanity.

3. Made a decision to turn our will and our lives over to the care of God as we understood Him.

4. Made a searching and fearless moral inventory of ourselves.

5. Admitted to God, to ourselves, and to another human being the exact nature of our wrongs.

6. Were entirely ready to have God remove all these defects of character.

7. Humbly asked Him to remove our shortcomings.

8. Made a list of all persons we had harmed, and became willing to make amends to them all.

9. Made direct amends to such people wherever possible, except when to do so would injure them or others.

10. Continued to take personal inventory, and when we were wrong, promptly admitted it.

11. Sought through prayer and meditation to improve our conscious contact with God, as we understood Him, praying only for knowledge of His will for us and the power to carry that out.

12. Having had a spiritual awakening as the result of these steps, we tried to carry this message to alcoholics, and to practice these principles in all our affairs.

Source. Reprinted with permission from A.A. World Services: *Twelve Steps and Twelve Traditions.* New York, A.A. World Services, Inc., 1981. The Twelve Steps are reprinted with permission of Alcoholics Anonymous World Services, Inc. ("A.A.W.S."). Permission to reprint the Twelve Steps does not mean that A.A.W.S. has reviewed or approved the contents of this publication, or that A.A. necessarily agrees with the views expressed herein. A.A. is a program of recovery from alcoholism only—use of the Twelve Steps in connection with programs and activities which are patterned after A.A., but which address other problems, or in any other non-A.A., does not imply otherwise.

Other 12-step programs focus on behavioral addictions, including Gamblers Anonymous, Sex and Love Addicts Anonymous, and Overeaters Anonymous.

The 12-step model has been helpful for family members of addicted individuals, with Al-Anon (for adults) and Alateen (for teenagers) being two of the most well-known 12-step programs to help family members.

Common Features of 12-Step Programs

Regardless of the focus of the 12-step program (e.g., AA, NA), the structure of the meetings shares many common features. Meetings often begin with a general statement of the definition of AA (from the Twelve Traditions), and it is common for members to introduce themselves by their first name and include in their introduction that they are "an alcoholic" or "an addict." Many meetings often end with the Serenity Prayer: "God, grant me the serenity to accept the things I cannot change, the courage to change the things I can, and the wisdom to know the difference."

It may be helpful to be able to educate patients that different types of meetings are available:

- *Open* meetings are those that are by definition open to any individual. A family member, or an interested health care professional wishing to learn more about how a 12-step meeting works, can attend an open meeting.
- *Closed* meetings are meetings specifically for individuals who identify as having the problem (e.g., alcoholism) or are questioning whether they have the problem.
- Other designations of meeting types include *speaker* meetings, during which an individual member presents his or her personal narrative; *step* meetings that focus on discussion of a specific step; and *discussion* meetings about a topic on which the group agrees.

AA and other 12-step programs incorporate the concept of sponsorship, in which the sponsor is designated to encourage and support a new member's desire for abstinence. The process of finding a sponsor may take some time, because a new member may wish to speak to several possible sponsors and find someone with whom he or she thinks he or she would be able to work well. Sponsors are not assigned by the group, but finding a sponsor is encouraged.

The sponsor and the newly sober member may

- Arrange to meet at meetings
- Talk on the telephone daily
- Meet independently to help the new member work on the steps, often focusing on Steps 4 and 5

In general, the rule is that a sponsor and sponsee should be of the same gender. Sponsorship is seen as an important aspect of the recovery process, not just in terms of providing support for the new member but also because the program emphasizes the importance of "carry[ing] this message to all alcoholics," as explained in Step 12 (Nace 2014). Physicians and other health care providers can help patients by explaining the sponsorship component of 12-step programs and inquiring at follow-up visits about whether the individual has yet found a sponsor.

History

AA was founded on June 10, 1935, by Dr. Bob Smith and Bill Wilson. The founders drew on several spiritual, philosophical, and psychological traditions as they developed AA, including teachings from the Oxford Group (an evangelical Christian group), the writings of William James, and the work of Carl Jung. There was also a significant contribution from Dr. William Silkworth, a neuropsychiatrist and medical director of the Charles B. Towns Hospital (a private alcohol treatment facility in New York City), who viewed alcoholism as a disease. Key events that led to the formation of the group included an experience of "spiritual awakening" that Bill Wilson had while being treated at the Towns Hospital (he saw a blinding white light and felt ecstatic while being treated with belladonna) and Bill Wilson's understanding, through personal experience, of the importance of communication among alcoholic persons as a means to facilitate sobriety (Kurtz 1991). Over time, AA has grown to have an estimated 2 million members worldwide (Nace 2014).

Subsequent 12-step groups were founded later: NA in the late 1940s, Cocaine Anonymous in 1982, and Marijuana Anonymous in 1989. Al-Anon was founded in 1951 by Lois Wilson, the wife of Bill Wilson, one of the founders of AA.

Spirituality

Historically, spirituality has been viewed as interchangeable with religiosity, or as an aspect within religiosity, and many people still might automatically link the concept of spirituality with religion. Interestingly, religion could be an example of one of the many ways in which people express their spirituality. *Religions* are institutions whose members adhere to doctrine and rituals, whereas *spirituality* is defined on an individual basis and requires subjective experience, which can be fluid over time. Spirituality involves "nonmaterial" issues that can be used to answer existential questions, such as the meaning of existence or the purpose of life. Spirituality is both something that an individual experiences and a process that he or she can pursue. For some, spirituality involves the supernatural or the sacred. For others, it can be related to natural phenomena or even considered within a scientific perspective. Some identify relationships or connections with others as their main spiritual focus.

Twelve-step programs, with their focus on the idea of a "higher power," emphasize the role of spirituality in recovery from addictive disorders; however, the concept of higher power and spirituality in AA and other 12-step programs can be interpreted widely according to an individual's beliefs and needs. These are not principles that connect specifically to one set of religious beliefs, although some individuals might define their higher power in terms of their already established religious beliefs or traditions. In 12-step programs, with regard to spirituality, what may be most important is that each member finds some way to define a higher power that aligns with a newly found meaning of life, one that will help sustain recovery.

Current research interest in the field of addiction focuses on developing a better understanding of spirituality, specifically how it pertains to addiction and recovery, because spiritual growth is such an essential element of the 12-step approach. Many argue that becoming more spiritual is an essential aspect of recovery, because AA specifically directs members to take on a more spiritual lifestyle. One of the co-founders of AA, Bill Wilson, wrote that people with addictions "have been not only mentally and physically ill, we have been spiritually sick. When the spiritual malady is overcome, we straighten out mentally and physically" (Alcoholics Anonymous 2001, p. 64). More broadly, spirituality is often considered related to psychological dimensions of health in general, such as hope, optimism, and inner peace (Sussman et al. 2013), and can incorporate elements of alternative medicine, such as meditation or prayer. Furthermore, strong evidence exists that spirituality protects against the development of substance use disorders and is associated with successful recovery. For example, religious people have consistently been shown to be less likely to become addicted to substances compared with people who are not religious, and AA members with more time sober have reported higher levels of spirituality (Miller and Bogenschutz 2007; Sussman et al. 2013; Treloar et al. 2014). However, it is not clear whether becoming spiritual facilitates recovery or whether recovery facilitates the development of spirituality. Depending on how narrowly or broadly spirituality is defined, this could be a bidirectional process.

Adapting spiritual beliefs and practicing spirituality can lead to a decrease in addictive behaviors, but various mediating factors could explain how spirituality can ultimately lead to a change in behavior. Some possibilities include

- Forming a relationship with a higher power
- Increasing psychological wellness
- Strengthening executive functioning
- Developing coping skills or improving social functioning
- Having a placebo effect

Although spirituality has been described as a multidimensional, latent, metaphysical construct that is not observable per se (and therefore more difficult to describe than more objective measures), several instruments have been developed to measure different aspects of spirituality (Galanter 2014). The very fact that spirituality is defined on an individual basis makes it difficult to study using traditional Western empirical methods. As a more scientific understanding of spirituality develops, the perceived gap between spiritual approaches and more traditional empirical approaches is likely to narrow.

It is important to maintain an open mind when talking with patients about spiritual issues, because spirituality has been associated with favorable substance abuse outcomes (see "Outcomes" section later in this chapter). Some examples of questions to begin to talk with patients about their spiritual beliefs are listed in Table 18–2. When assessing spirituality, it is important to consider various factors that can contribute to a person's spiritual beliefs, such as

- Cultural heritage
- Societal norms
- Religious upbringing

Furthermore, taking a nonjudgmental approach might help uncover any resistance patients might have to discussing spirituality.

When working with patients with substance use disorders, it may be beneficial for a health care provider to have some sense of his or her own spiritual beliefs, in order to more effectively discuss spiritual issues and questions with patients. The provider should be open to the spiritual beliefs of patients and supportive of the patient's development of a sense of spirituality, because for many individuals, finding meaning in life and taking on a more spiritual lifestyle can lead to a decrease in addictive behaviors.

TABLE 18–2. Questions to consider asking patients to assess for spirituality

Do you consider yourself to be a spiritual person?

Do you practice spirituality or participate in any spiritual events?

Do you meditate or pursue spiritual experiences?

Have you ever thought about the meaning (or purpose) of your life?

What are the things that give your life meaning?

Source. Adapted from Sussman et al. 2013.

Outcomes

Some patients have come into contact with 12-step programs in the community even before they engage in any other type of treatment program, and providers commonly recommend AA or other 12-step programs. Participation in AA is associated with increased abstinence, with studies showing small to moderate effect sizes. Furthermore, abstinence is even more likely should the person commit to and practice the behaviors prescribed by AA (Tonigan and Forcehimes 2011).

Twelve-step facilitation, a therapy designed to help patients actively engage in 12-step programs in addition to accepting the need for abstinence, has been shown to result in better outcomes when compared with no treatment and was equally as effective as other treatment modalities such as cognitive-behavioral therapy (Nace 2014). It is not clear as to which of the 12 steps might be more beneficial and how long such possible benefit persists, although it is worth considering that addiction is a chronic condition for which long-term treatment is often most effective. Possible reasons that patients benefit from 12-step programs include the following (Nace 2014):

- Participation in the group process
- Maturation of the "self"
- Interaction with empathetic peers
- Development of spirituality (as discussed earlier)

Having a sponsor was associated with increased frequency of meeting attendance and with positive outcomes with regard to reduced drinking. Finally, in terms of being a sponsor, some evidence has shown that helping other members was associated with a higher quality of life and duration of time sober (Tonigan and Forcehimes 2011).

How to Incorporate 12-Step Meetings Into a Patient's Treatment

Because 12-step program engagement can potentially be a very positive predictor of success for patients struggling with addictions, health care providers should be familiar with the basic goals, structure, and philosophy of these meetings so that they can recommend this option to appropriate patients who might derive significant benefit. Table 18–3 includes suggestions for how health care providers can help engage their patients in 12-step program participation.

Individuals often report that they do not like AA if they did not feel comfortable at the first meeting they attended; therefore, it can be helpful to provide some anticipatory guid-

TABLE 18–3. Ways to encourage patient participation in 12-step meetings

Encourage patients to try multiple meetings.

Encourage patients to find a home group.

Have a list handy of local meeting times and locations (often easily found online).

Some areas have a hotline number that is staffed by 12-step members (especially Alcoholics Anonymous); ask the patient to call with you while in your office.

Be prepared to offer education about the ways in which "God" and "spirituality" can be broadly interpreted for individuals concerned about the potential religious focus of 12-step meetings.

Consider attending an open meeting to gain firsthand experience about meetings, in order to be able to better counsel your patients about what to expect.

ance for the patient, explaining that finding a meeting in which the individual feels comfortable may take some trial and error. AA meetings can be comprised of different populations of people, and some meetings may be more diverse than others. Considering this variety, a patient may find a specific meeting in which he or she feels more comfortable. Furthermore, it can be helpful to encourage patients to find a home group (or a group in which he or she feels comfortable, would attend weekly, and possibly taking on some of the responsibilities of running the meeting, such as being a greeter, setting up chairs, or making coffee). Developing individual connections to others in the home group can be an important component of developing a support system for the newly sober individual.

Some patients may express reservations about the perceived religious focus of AA and other 12-step meetings. It can be helpful to discuss with patients that there can be multiple interpretations of "higher power." Many individuals find it helpful to think of their higher power as the AA group itself. Some alcoholic individuals who are agnostic or atheist have suggested, with good humor, that for them the God referred to in the Twelve Steps is the "Group of Drunks." Whatever is identified as the higher power, the important message, central to AA, is that the member accepts that he or she is not

God. The emphasis on fellowship and the interpersonal connectedness that stems from this may be helpful factors to emphasize for patients who are reluctant to try meetings because of concerns about the religious focus. As Kurtz (1991) says in his book on the history of AA, "The fulfilling of the implications of being not-God, the living out of the connectedness with others that comes about from the alcoholic's very limitation, is the story of Alcoholics Anonymous" (p. 3). That said, some AA meetings are specifically for atheist and agnostic individuals ("Agnostic AA" meetings).

Some patients, as well as some health care providers, have concerns about whether treatment with medications— psychiatric or otherwise—will be criticized in a 12-step program. The official AA position about medications is that the individual and the physician should decide if the use of medications is appropriate. Although this is the AA position, individual members, including patients' sponsors, might have their own views and might even try to influence the patient. The pamphlet "The AA Member—Medications and Other Drugs" (Alcoholics Anonymous 2011) clarifies the AA position and emphasizes that even though "it is generally accepted that the misuse of prescription medication and other drugs can threaten the achievement and maintenance of sobriety," this risk may be mitigated by emphasizing that the AA member's treatment should be guided by a qualified physician ("no AA member should 'play doctor'"), and the patient should be honest with the physician about his or her sobriety, as well as about any misuse of prescription medications.

KEY POINTS

Twelve-step programs are nonprofessional, self-supporting, apolitical programs that are open to anyone who wants to stop drinking or using drugs.

Members of 12-step programs are encouraged to attend meetings and to work through a series of 12 steps, often with the aid of a sponsor—a more senior member of the same gender who has achieved sobriety for at least 1 year.

Spirituality, which may or may not encompass an individual's belief in God or connection to organized religion, provides a meaningful sense of something outside the self and is often an important part of recovery from substance use disorders.

Because participation in 12-step programs is associated with positive substance abuse outcomes, possibly by fostering spiritual growth, clinicians are encouraged to have a basic understanding of spirituality and 12-step programs and should consider recommending participation to appropriate patients.

References

Alcoholics Anonymous: Alcoholics Anonymous: The Story of How Many Thousands of Men and Women Have Recovered From Alcoholism, 4th Edition. New York, AA World Services, 2001

Alcoholics Anonymous: The AA Member—Medications and Other Drugs. New York, Alcoholics Anonymous World Services, 2011

Alcoholics Anonymous: Alcoholics Anonymous Web site, 2015. Available at: http://www.aa.org. Accessed January 24, 2015.

Galanter M: Spirituality in the recovery process, in The ASAM Principles of Addiction Medicine, 5th Edition. Edited by Ries R. Philadelphia, PA, Lippincott Williams & Wilkins, 2014, pp 1060–1063

Kurtz E: Not-God: A History of Alcoholics Anonymous. Center City, MN, Hazelden, 1991

Miller WR, Bogenschutz MP: Spirituality and addiction. South Med J 100(4):433–436, 2007 17458418

Nace EP: Twelve-step programs in addiction recovery, in The ASAM Principles of Addiction Medicine, 5th Edition. Edited by Ries R. Philadelphia, PA, Lippincott Williams & Wilkins, 2014, pp 1033–1042

Sussman S, Milam J, Arpawong TE, et al: Spirituality in addictions treatment: wisdom to know…what it is. Subst Use Misuse 48(12):1203–1217, 2013 24041182

Tonigan JS, Forcehimes AA: Religiousness, spirituality, and addiction: an evidence-based review, in Addiction Medicine. Edited by Johnson BA. New York, Springer, 2011, pp 1217–1235

Treloar HR, Dubreuil ME, Miranda R Jr: Spirituality and treatment of addictive disorders. R I Med J 97(3):36–38, 2014 24596929

CHAPTER 19

Mindfulness and Mentalization

MARYN SLOANE, M.D.

CRAVING is a compulsive or pathological desire to use or experience the effects of a substance and can be experienced as

- Intrusive thoughts
- An affective state
- An impulsive drive
- A bodily sensation
- Quite simply, "wanting"

Craving may be perceived so intensely as to sabotage short-term recovery and significantly interfere with sustained recovery. The significance of craving as a predictor for relapse has been widely appreciated by researchers, clinicians, and patients alike for decades. However, comprehensive and unified models for craving have not been fully conceptualized or integrated. Furthermore, the relation between craving and relapse has been difficult to quantify. Despite this, it is widely accepted that craving is both a significant symptom of disease and an obstacle to remission. Therefore, this is a critical target of treatment.

Craving can be conceptualized from its biological, psychic, social, and behavioral underpinnings. Each of these concepts may have unique pharmacological, psychological, and behavioral treatment modalities associated with them. Viewed from an affective perspective, craving and relapse are a result of positive associations of the effects of a drug with use or, more frequently, are associated with the desire to avoid negative affective states. Cognitively speaking, craving and relapse may be conceptualized as being driven by overlearned patterns of thought and emotion, with use characterized as repetitive, automatic, and engaging little conscious thought. Biologically, craving and relapse may result from conditioned responses to drug-related cues, a disturbance of homeostatic regulation in neurotransmitters, or physiological withdrawal.

It is commonly accepted that effective treatment strategies for addictive disorders must address all of the neurobiological, cognitive, and affective bases of the disease. Drawing on both cognitive-behavioral and psychodynamic therapeutic traditions, mindfulness-based and mentalization-based treatments for addictive disorders both offer a perspective on these known foundations for relapse and craving, as well as a promising focus of intervention. These separate entities share roots in the treatment of borderline personality disorder and are characterized by the favoring of present attention over reflexive reactivity and the abandonment of restrictive patterns of thoughts and feelings. Developed in concert, these practices are thought to be synergistic.

Clinicians agree that the treatment of drug addictions must offer an encompassing range of services—medical, social, and psychological. The place of psychotherapeutic work is indisputably central, because it is directed at changing the psychic functioning of the patient. It is assumed that this happens through a gradual process that deepens the patient's understanding of the place of addiction in his or her life.

Mindfulness

WHAT IS MINDFULNESS?

Mindfulness is a term that has been made popular through the ancient writings and practices of Eastern Buddhism. Its simple translation is "bare attention." Jon Kabat-Zinn (2003, p. 145), the psychologist credited with early integration of mindfulness-based interventions into modern clinical practice, defines *mindfulness* as "the awareness that emerges through paying attention, on purpose, in the present moment, and non-judgmentally to the unfolding of experience." The Buddhist perspective espoused by the teaching of the Four Noble Truths is the desire for and separation from that which we find pleasing—craving and attachment, the root of all human suffering. Hence, cessation of suffering comes through relinquishment of craving. Craving is relinquished through "seeing with wisdom" that feelings are not intrinsically pleasant or painful but merely *are*. This perspective is achieved through the individual's constant awareness of his or her feelings as they arise and meditative practices that culminate in the correct control of the mind and behavior.

The practice has been venerated by followers of the Buddha as a means of interrupting what would otherwise become an insufferable repetitive cycle of action and reaction, born from disappointing attachments that further prevent our abilities to appreciate true perspective. It is taught that our attachments and reactions become the progenitors of our distress and not the events themselves. Reactions may become conditioned and unalterable. Viewed from this perspective, craving may be described as an effort to avoid suffering by clinging to positive states (chasing the next high) or to avoid a negative state (as an escape from depression or anxiety).

Mindfulness practice is composed of two basic tenets:

1. An individual being vividly aware of his or her current experience: This draws an exception to the idea that in an individual's usual state of mental awareness, the mind operates in a reflexive and automatic fashion in which most experiences go by mindlessly unrecognized and unacknowledged.
2. An individual fully accepting his or her current experience: The individual becomes free from reactivity or judgment toward any particular thoughts or experiences.

Mindfulness in practice involves training in the individual's ability to observe craving as it is perceived, but more importantly, to recognize it as a temporary and passing state of affliction: to learn to experience a sensation without reaction or judgment. In doing so, the individual begins to recognize that all affective states are temporary. The mindfulness practitioner learns over time and repeated exposures that the cognitive and affective response to the craving causes distress and not the craving itself.

HOW DO WE DEVELOP MINDFULNESS?

The capacity for mindfulness is a quality all humans possess and enlist for use, sometimes unintentionally—the ability to override the din of our ever-present mindless noise and instead focus awareness completely on the experience of the current moment. To learn to harness and direct this capacity, a combination of guided instruction and personal practice generally is sufficient. The skill is then best developed through repeated practice. Activities that foster mindfulness may be

- Formal, such as yoga or meditation
- Informal, such as mindful stretching on waking or mindful eating

Activities that foster mindfulness may be interspersed into daily activities, or mindfulness may be an activity itself for which time is set aside within the daily routine.

At its most basic level, mindfulness may be fostered by engaging in any activity that shifts the mind from wandering to an active and aware state. Capacity to concentrate is developed by bringing attention to an object repeatedly and bringing attention back yet again if the mind wanders or becomes distracted. It can be as simple as noticing how the chair feels underneath you when you are seated. The breath is commonly used as the object of focus and awareness. The practice then extends to include the awareness and acknowledgment of all thoughts and physical and emotional sensations. The practice of focusing and then sustaining attention on the current moment is thought to enhance the ability to notice and to be able to interrupt behavioral patterns.

MINDFULNESS IN CLINICAL PRACTICE

The development of mindfulness as a therapeutic technique was first used with patients who had painful and chronic conditions in the hospital setting. Traditionally, mindfulness is fostered through personal meditative practice. In the Western clinical domain, mindfulness-based treatments have been packaged to be delivered to groups of patients in programs that consist of multiple skills and psychoeducational training sessions. Patients are expected to practice and incorporate the learned skills outside of session. Research has confirmed beneficial effects of mindfulness-based treatments for a wide variety of medical and psychiatric disorders with formats that have been adapted for the specific disorder they are designed to treat. Within psychotherapy, mindfulness-based programs have included

- Mindfulness-based stress reduction
- Mindfulness-based eating awareness training
- Mindfulness-based cognitive therapy
- Acceptance and commitment therapy (ACT)
- Dialectical behavioral therapy (DBT)
- Mindfulness-based relapse prevention (MBRP)

MINDFULNESS-BASED STRESS REDUCTION

Mindfulness-based stress reduction was developed and popularized by psychologist Jon Kabat-Zinn. It was adapted from Eastern Zen traditions and formatted for use with hospitalized patients who had pain, anxiety, depression, or terminal illness. Although mindfulness is culturally and traditionally a solitary practice with roots that seem almost at odds with Western medicine, it has since been separated from its Eastern origins and framed into a group practice that is offered extensively across the United States in a variety of settings, including hospitals, clinics, assisted living facilities, community centers, prisons, and workplaces.

The program follows a manualized format of eight weekly group sessions during which patients are provided psychoeducation on the nature of stress and then receive guided instruction on specific mindfulness and meditative techniques, such as a "lying-down body scan" or "loving-kindness meditation." Groups are relatively large (30–40 people), and the course is time-limited. Instructors are expected to be practitioners themselves. Patients are advised to continue to practice what has been presented in an ongoing manner outside of the sessions to achieve maximum benefit.

Mindfulness-based trainings as an adjunct to traditional medical treatment for many disorders have increased dramatically in the past 30 years. In a variety of disorders—immunological, autoimmune, pain, endocrine, dermatological—benefits were measured beyond subjective anxiety and depression. Outcomes of small yet descriptive studies have been undertaken and/or reviewed by the Center for Mindfulness in Medicine, Health Care, and Society and by its Stress Reduction Clinic in an attempt to characterize and qualify the healing and restorative effects of mindfulness in clinical medical settings. Among these, a blinded and randomized study of 37 patients with psoriasis reported a fourfold rate of skin improvement in meditators as compared with nonmeditators (Kabat-Zinn et al. 1998). In another study, 10 prostate cancer patients with metastatic disease and rising prostate-specific antigen (PSA) values were trained in mindfulness-based stress reduction. Investigators found that the rate of rise of PSA significantly decreased in 8 of the 10 patients, thus delaying the PSA doubling time by 11 months (Kabat-Zinn 2003).

Investigations such as these illuminate the promise that mindfulness-based adjunctive interventions may have in the care of patients and in the treatment of specific diseases. Mindfulness-based stress reduction program manuals and workbooks are widely available, as are instructional recordings of the meditative practices.

Free resources, including audio files available for download, may be found at the following Web sites: The Free Mindfulness Project (www.freemindfulness.org) and the Center for Mindfulness in Medicine, Health Care, and Society (www.umassmed.edu/cfm).

MINDFULNESS-BASED EATING AWARENESS TRAINING

Eating with awareness can be undertaken formally as a group practice or informally incorporated into the eating of meals. The purpose of this exercise is to develop awareness of and appreciation for the depth of sensation that occurs through eating; it was designed to help treat binge-eating disorder and compulsive or mindless eating.

When incorporated informally, mindful eating may be as simple an exercise as putting your fork down between bites to allow a moment for your focus and attention to recalibrate. A format developed by psychologist Jean Kristeller called MB-EAT uses more formal practice and is designed to help those who have eating disorders, along with co-occurring deficits such as poor sensitivity to satiety, prominent guilt, disconnection from internal awareness that may lead to overeating, cues that trigger eating apart from hunger such as anxiety and depression, and the sense of being out of control that often accompanies binge eating.

MINDFULNESS-BASED COGNITIVE THERAPY

Mindfulness-based cognitive therapy was developed by Zindel Segal, Mark Williams, and John Teasdale for relapsing depression. It combines the practice of mindfulness meditation along with the practical skills of cognitive therapy. Cognitive therapy is explained in greater detail in Chapter 15, "Cognitive-Behavioral Therapy."

ACCEPTANCE AND COMMITMENT THERAPY

Developed by Steven C. Hayes, Kelly G. Wilson, and Kirk Strosahl, ACT was first implemented in the 1980s and has since been formally manualized. It is composed of six core processes that are based on mindfulness principles and behavioral activation:

1. Accepting what may be uncomfortable experiences, thoughts, or feelings to maintain flexibility
2. Engaging in cognitive defusion of automatic uncomfortable thoughts (enabling the individual to observe them, not add value to them)
3. Being present; to voluntarily direct attention wholly to the moment, not automatically focusing on the past or future
4. Using the individual self as context; always checking and rechecking assumptions about personal experiences
5. Identifying the values that are important to the individual and to the kind of person he or she would like to be
6. Being committed to achieving those values

ACT is delivered in individual therapy sessions, small groups, large groups, workshops, and books or other media. The therapeutic interventions might be provided through psychoeducation, dialogue, visualization exercises, or behavioral homework. They are selected from a broad arsenal of ACT-elaborated exercises intended to match the decided-on treatment goals. Exercises are intended to be flexible and adaptive for a wide range of clinical sessions. Length of treatment will vary depending on preferences and needs of the patient and therapist.

DIALECTICAL BEHAVIORAL THERAPY

DBT is a didactic therapy regimen, in part for mindfulness skills training. It was developed by Marsha Linehan, both a psychologist and a person with borderline personality disorder. She successfully used the model on herself in her own struggle, which she revealed many years after its introduction. The principles and interventions are similar to other cognitive and behavioral treatments, yet are adapted for patients who may be more limited in their attention and psychical resources (as are those who have moderate to severe personality disorders). Mindfulness training is not expected

to be formalized into practice by the patients, and the therapist is not required to practice. Exercises are simplified and
focus on learning how to observe and describe rather than on
judging or automatically reacting.

DBT has been associated with

- An increased awareness of the processes that lead up to
  an action
- Decreases in impulsive behavior
- Greater acceptance of negative emotions that formerly
  would have triggered impulsive actions

MINDFULNESS-BASED RELAPSE PREVENTION

Relapse is highly prevalent following substance abuse treatment. MBRP is a psychosocial- and group-based aftercare
treatment developed by Dr. Alan Marlatt in collaboration
with his colleagues; it draws on his vast breadth of work on
the effects of transcendental meditation, spanning the 1970s
into the twenty-first century. MBSRP is an outpatient intervention that marries cognitive-behavioral techniques with
training in mindfulness meditation practice. There is no one
manualized technical approach to this intervention, and various training options are available to suit the specific patient
populations the clinician serves.

The mindfulness-based approach is especially well suited
to not only the prevention of relapse but to addiction in general. If addiction is a frantic effort to avoid uncomfortable affective states—and the reflexive responses to such avoidance
through the impulsive use of mind-altering chemical substances, mindfulness is the antithetical alternative to how an
individual might respond to these thoughts and resulting behaviors. Increased awareness—rather than the dulling of
awareness—is the key to the success of this model. While the
individual increases awareness of the present moment, the si-
multaneous ability to respond more skillfully and less reflexively is developed. These interventions also stress developing
individuals' compassion toward themselves and their experiences, increasing awareness of personal triggers, changing
their relationship to discomfort in general, and building a life
that helps to promote recovery. Research that includes brain
imaging is currently underway to identify what is hypothesized to be identifiable reparative changes in the brain systems
that become damaged in response to addiction and addictive

behaviors. MBRP has been shown to be an effective aftercare approach for individuals recently completing intensive substance abuse treatment, in reducing subsequent substance use and teaching alternative responses to discomfort while lessening the conditioned response of craving.

SUMMARY

There is commonality in all of these mindfulness-based interventions. That is, in every mindful moment there exists a choice point—an opportunity to do things differently and less destructively. This is as true, for example, in the engagement of destructive eating behaviors; in malefic impulsive behaviors in personal and professional relationships, which divide instead of bridge connections; and in reflexively giving into craving through the use of chemical substances in response to negative affective states. All of these mindfulness-based techniques serve to widen the space between thought and behavior, enhance the individual's comfort with and acceptance of his or her experience within that space, and develop his or her skillful awareness in order to make thoughtful and purposeful, positive choices in response.

MINDFULNESS IN PATIENTS WITH SUBSTANCE USE DISORDERS

Within the field of addiction, mindfulness-based skills training has been specifically adapted for treatment of substance use disorders. When combined with relapse prevention, it is known as mindfulness-based relapse prevention. Participation in mindfulness-based treatments for substance use disorders has been shown to result in

- Decreases in craving and substance use
- A decreased association between depressive symptoms and craving

Relapse prevention strategies enhance individuals' coping and self-efficacy and challenge automatic expectations that a substance will have a desirable effect (see Chapter 16, "Relapse Prevention," for further discussion). Mindful meditation facilitates an alternative way for individuals to manage themselves in a situation that may place them at high risk for relapse. With this coping strategy, the individual learns to be aware, accepting, and nonpartisan to powerful feelings, thoughts, and sensations that would typically result in relapse (especially craving and physiological withdrawal).

Another element of traditional relapse prevention training is the recognition and development of awareness for drug-related cues that serve as warning signs for pending relapse. For example, individuals in recovery often come into the company of a substance-using acquaintance or find themselves in a location they associate with prior substance use. Mindfulness training teaches them a new method of relating to these high-risk situations: to develop awareness and to observe and accept reactions without allowing these to drive a behavioral response. This learned pattern of mindful behavior then becomes the welcomed alternative to relapse in the face of high-risk exposures. The ability to tolerate high-risk situations and maintain abstinence fosters self-efficacy. In the end, this form of positive reinforcement becomes more validating than the effects of the substance.

Mentalization

WHAT IS MENTALIZATION?

Mentalization is defined as "the capacity to think about mental states as separate from, yet potentially causing, actions." It is the process that "allows us to perceive and interpret human behavior in terms of intentional mental states" (Bateman and Fonagy 2004, p. 36). Mentalization refers to the moment-to-moment dynamic representation we each have of ourselves and those with whom we interact, which is a product of needs, desires, feelings, beliefs, goals, purposes, and reasons. Like mindfulness, mentalization also highlights the significance of focused awareness for what is actually experienced over judgments and reactivity—yet it also goes beyond this, asking the individual to formulate an idea about the mental states of himself or herself and others.

Failure to develop the capacity to mentalize results in a variety of disorders and problem behaviors. Appropriately elaborated, mentalization is associated with an individual's

- Ability to perceive himself or herself and situations from multiple vantage points
- Increased capacity to problem-solve and manage stress
- Mastery over his or her own behavior

Furthermore, failure to mentalize in a relationship can lead to an individual's

- Repetitive maladaptive interactions
- Attribution of his or her perhaps faulty feelings onto another
- Failure to see himself or herself or interactions realistically

Addiction may be conceived as failure of the capacity to mentalize that arises either

- Directly from the use of substances; or
- When a vulnerable person without the capacity to mentalize is exposed to stress and begins using substances as a means to cope.

HOW DO WE DEVELOP MENTALIZATION?

At its most basic level, mentalization in a psychotherapeutic interaction is simply identifying and labeling feelings. This is a concept known as *mentalized affectivity* and refers to the uniquely human skill to "feel and think about feeling" simultaneously (Bateman and Fonagy 2004). Attachment is seen as the main factor governing the development of mentalization, wherein the mother-infant bond provides the essential framework for a human to begin to develop this skill. An inability to mentalize ultimately leaves an individual powerless to exercise control over his or her own affective states. However, identifying and expressing emotions enable an individual to control the duration and intensity of these emotions without resorting to impulsive means in order to avoid them entirely. The use of substances can be one type of such impulsive means, in which a person self-medicates to diminish or avoid emotions.

Unlike more traditional analytic therapies, mentalization-based treatment focuses on easily accessible content and on the immediate interaction and alliance between patient and therapist. The therapist is active in the treatment role, encouraging attachment and hence a "turning on" of the activation system, which then makes it possible for patient and therapist to explore deficits in mentalization. This secure attachment and safe exploration enable restructuring of mentalization capacity.

MENTALIZATION IN CLINICAL PRACTICE

Mentalization-based treatment, a type of psychodynamically oriented psychotherapy, was developed by the psychologist Peter Fonagy and the psychiatrist Anthony Bateman in the 2000s, although its theoretical roots go back to the early 1990s. It borrows from the principles of currently available therapeutic interventions for personality disorders. Like DBT, treatment focuses on the moment-to-moment mental state of the patient. The goal of therapy is to help the patient to understand, coherently integrate, and accurately represent internal mental states and thus to improve the ability to mentalize.

Mentalization-based treatment differs from other insight-oriented psychotherapies such as psychoanalysis, in that subconscious and unconscious conflicts are not worthwhile or desirable targets for exploration. Present awareness, thoughts, and feelings are of main therapeutic import. Also, unlike psychoanalysis, in which the therapist maintains calm neutrality, the therapist stance in mentalization-based treatment is caring and emotionally invested (much like the integrative and interpersonal approaches to psychotherapy). This approach as described by Bateman and Fonagy is well structured and focused on fostering the attachment between patient and therapist, and the immediate interaction (transference) between patient and therapist guides the direction of treatment.

The essential features of the treatment as formally prescribed by Bateman and Fonagy include alternating group and individual psychotherapy sessions twice weekly. The purpose of alternating sessions is to provide balance: the attachment activation work accomplished in an individual session can be tempered by a group session, and the intensity of the group can be ameliorated by the relatively more attentive environment of the individual session. In this way, the activation of attachment is carefully monitored alongside the development of mentalizing skills. To enhance mentalization skills, the mentalization-based treatment therapist specifically aims to

- Provide a structure and framework that is both interested and available but not intrusive
- Bridge the gap between the patient's inner experience and how it is represented in order to facilitate intentional over impulsive behaviors

- Facilitate the identification and understanding of current emotional states experienced by the patient and help to put them into context
- Be consistently mindful of the patient's deficits

MENTALIZATION IN PATIENTS WITH SUBSTANCE USE DISORDERS

Generally speaking, psychotherapy in a substance-abusing population is considered tenuous. Issues such as treatment retention, inability to manage states of frustration, and potential to relapse as a means to cope with negative affective states render traditional psychodynamically based psychotherapies poorly tolerated or ineffective. In contrast to cognitive, behavioral, motivational, and mindfulness-based treatments, which may be effectively and appropriately initiated in a variety of treatment stages and settings, mentalization-based treatment is not a treatment for someone newly sober. As with other psychodynamic therapies, it is recommended that a patient be stably sober before mentalization-based treatment is undertaken. The required length of sober time varies from patient to patient, although 3 months of abstinence is generally agreed on as a good estimate. For opioid-addicted patients, medication-assisted treatment in the form of buprenorphine or methadone is recommended as an adjunct to mentalization-based treatment.

Mentalization is the individual's ability to recognize subjective mental states in himself or herself and in others and appreciate that others' mental states may not correlate with what is observed. This ability is thought to derive from having secure attachments as a child. If mentalization is not developed appropriately, the result is affective instability, impulsive behaviors, and unstable relationships later in life.

KEY POINTS

The pathological compulsion to use a substance, known as craving, has complex and interwoven neurobiological, cognitive, behavioral, affective, social, and environmental underpinnings. The most successful treatments for mitigating relapse and sustaining remission will attempt to address all of these underlying components.

Mindfulness may be defined as paying attention to the present on purpose, moment by moment, and without judgment. It may be refined through formal or informal daily practice and has been adapted into various interventions shown to be of benefit in both medical and psychiatric disease.

For the treatment of addiction, mindfulness-based relapse prevention cultivates mindful awareness for cues, triggers, and responses to craving; increases ability to tolerate the discomfort associated with craving; and helps the patient acquire nonreactive behaviors over former patterns that served to relieve distress temporarily but led to negative outcomes (such as relapse).

Addiction may be seen as a failure in the ability to mentalize or a desire to avoid mentalizing. Mentalization-based treatment aims to provide the secure attachment whereby a patient may explore the world of his or her own mind and that of others (the therapist). By doing so, the patient may then become fully aware of and tolerant of his or her own mental states.

Mindfulness-based and mentalization-based treatments for addictive disorders are each useful in their own right, yet they are also synergistic interventions that target the well-described "root causes" of craving and relapse. Both are characterized by the individual's emphasis on attention to the present moment, developing awareness for his or her own thoughts and behaviors, and decreasing mindless emotionality and reflexive reactivity, with the goal of freeing him or her from the restrictive patterns of thoughts, feelings, and behaviors that perpetuate addiction.

References

Bateman A, Fonagy P: Psychotherapy for Borderline Personality Disorder: Mentalization-Based Treatment. New York, Oxford University Press, 2004

Kabat-Zinn J: Mindfulness-based interventions in context: past, present, and future. Clinical Psychology: Science and Practice 10(2):144–156, 2003

Kabat-Zinn J, Wheeler E, Light T, et al: Influence of a mindfulness meditation-based stress reduction intervention on rates of skin clearing in patients with moderate to severe psoriasis undergoing phototherapy (UVB) and photochemotherapy (PUVA). Psychosom Med 60(5):625–632, 1998 9773769

CHAPTER 20

Diet and Exercise

SONYA LAZAREVIC, M.D., M.S.

ALEX ZAPHIRIS, M.D., M.S.

AN integrative approach to treating substance use disorders is a rapidly expanding area of interest in the outpatient and rehabilitation settings. Growth in this area is matched both by practitioners and by patients who seek complementary therapies to relieve suffering or to provide assistance when conventional treatment falls short (Barnes et al. 2004).

Principles of Integrative Addiction Treatment

Based on the principles of integrative medicine as defined by the Arizona Center for Integrative Medicine, integrative addiction treatment

- Provides relationship-centered care
- Integrates conventional and complementary and alternative medicine methods of treatment and prevention
- Uses natural, less invasive interventions when possible
- Engages the whole person—mind, body, and spirit— as well as the community
- Focuses attention on lifestyle choices for prevention and maintenance of health
- Maintains that healing is always possible even when curing is not

Diet (Food Choices)

The foci of this chapter, diet and exercise, are central components of lifestyle counseling when treating addictions with integrative approaches. When evaluating a patient's diet, it is useful to explore the following internal and external influencing factors affecting food choices:

- Financial limitations
- Access to quality food
- Eating habits of others living in the home
- Medical needs
- Beliefs, culture, and habits around food
- Patient's understanding of the relation between food choices and health

Food is an integral aspect of individual (or family) identity and may represent the language in which people express themselves or interact with others. Some patients may be able to afford organic vegetables, whereas others may live in a food-insecure household, without reliable access to a sufficient quantity of affordable, nutritious food.

Recommending that a patient "go on a diet" tends to connote weight loss or restriction or denial of some kind. Alternatively, we suggest inviting a nonjudgmental conversation about "food and nutritional choices." Exploring nutritional habits could be initiated through discussion guided by a food journal:

- Ask the patient to journal all meals, snacks, and beverages (including soda, juice, coffee) consumed over 1 week, broken down into morning, midday, and evening.
- Invite a discussion around the experience of keeping a food journal, and discuss how, why, and when choices were made.

The clinician may evaluate and educate a patient through different stages of recovery (postacute withdrawal; early recovery: 3–9 months; sustained recovery: 12 or more months). To assess how dietary choices and habits are affected by substance use:

- Obtain a baseline pattern of nutritional habits
- Ascertain dietary habits during periods of use
- After use, determine whether this pattern changes and, if so, how
- Assess eating habits 1 week after last use compared with 2 or 4 months after use
- Identify food choices during prior episodes of sobriety

The **anti-inflammatory diet** is an excellent nutritional recommendation for the person in recovery to help improve overall health and support recovery from addiction. The anti-inflammatory diet emphasizes eating vegetables, whole grains, and quality meats and fats that are nutrient dense; it also limits processed and packaged foods that contain poor-quality fats, sugar, chemicals, and few nutrients. An overview of the anti-inflammatory diet is included in Table 20–1.

A **protein-rich diet** also should be considered for patients in recovery. Animal and human studies find that malnourishment increases sensitivity to addiction and that patients with opioid and alcohol use disorders specifically have protein malnutrition. It is known that people under emotional or physical stress require more protein than usual. Table 20–2 lists examples of protein sources.

TABLE 20–1. Principles of the anti-inflammatory diet

Eat multiple servings of vegetables daily, including those of different colors.

Avoid foods in packaging (these tend to have higher amount of preservatives, additives, and chemicals).

Avoid foods with hormones or antibiotics.

Select fresh fruits and vegetables, which are preferred over frozen fruits and vegetables, and select frozen fruits and vegetables over canned. When possible, select seasonal produce.

Read all labels.

Monitor (likely increase) fiber intake—beans, whole grains, vegetables, and fruits.

Monitor fat intake: 25%–35% of diet.
- Maintain ratio of 1:2:1 of saturated to monounsaturated to polyunsaturated fat.
- Limit saturated fats, such as in red meat and dairy.
- Increase mono- and polyunsaturated fats found in canola oil, olive oil, nuts, avocado, and fatty fish.
- Limit trans fats such as those found in fried foods, bakery goods, and partially hydrogenated vegetable oils.
- Increase omega-3 fatty acids.
  - Flax seed (2 tbsp/day or 1 tbsp oil/day), walnuts, pumpkin seeds, hen eggs
  - Fatty fish (salmon, lake trout, sardines, tuna); avoid farm-raised salmon

Limit sugar intake (6 tsp maximum daily).
- Reduce refined sugars, white flours, soda, and fruit juice.
- Alternatively, use (in moderation) fruits, honey, brown sugar, and maple syrup.

Limit salt intake (1 tsp maximum daily).

Choose foods low on the glycemic index.

Reduce or eliminate caffeinated beverages.

TABLE 20–2. Examples of protein sources

Food	Amount of protein
Egg	6 g
Lean meat, fish, poultry	25–30 g per 3.5 oz
Tofu	20 g per cup
Tempeh	30 g per cup
Milk	8–9 g per cup
Yogurt	8–10 g per cup
Cheddar/jack cheese	7 g per oz
Cottage cheese	28 g per cup
Nuts and seeds	2–3 g per tbsp
Beans, cooked	15 g per cup

Source. Adapted from U.S. Department of Agriculture nutrient database.

NUTRIENT DEFICIENCY AND REPLACEMENT

NUTRITION AND OPIOID USE

A limited number of studies have examined the relation between nutrition and opioid addiction.

- Males with chronic opiate addiction tend to replace foods rich in protein and fat with foods rich in sucrose and poor in vitamins and minerals (Morabia et al. 1989).
- Of the heroin-addicted individuals in withdrawal, 74% had clinical evidence of nutrient deficiency, and more than 60% presented with multiple deficiencies and malnutrition (Nazrul Islam et al. 2002).
- Use of neurotransmitter precursors in acute opioid withdrawal resulted in fewer withdrawal symptoms, less insomnia, and improved mood symptoms compared with placebo. Study details are as follows (Chen et al. 2012):
  - Study protocol:
    1) In the morning, L-tyrosine 50 mg/kg/day (for 140-lb individual=3,000 mg/day) and lecithin 1,200 mg/day, containing phosphatidylcholine 210 mg;
    2) 1.5 hours before bed, L-glutamine 50 mg/kg/day (for 140-lb individual=3,000 mg/day), 5-hydroxytryptophan 400 mg/day (undivided dose) total.

Diet and Exercise

- Study duration was only 7 days, but regimen may be beneficial for a longer duration.
- Most common adverse symptom was nausea, which may be related to withdrawal and not supplements.

- Opioid withdrawal is associated with oxidative stress and decreased antioxidants. The more severe the opioid dependence, the greater the oxidative stress. Studies of high-dose oral vitamin C showed that vitamin C blocks opioid receptors in the brain and attenuates withdrawal symptoms. Protocol for one study is shown as follows (Evangelou et al. 2000):
  - Dosage: ascorbic acid 300 mg/kg/day, supplemented with vitamin E (5 mg/kg/day) in divided doses every 2–3 hours during waking hours.
  - Continue for 1 month; may cause diarrhea.

NUTRITION AND ALCOHOL USE

The short- and long-term toxic effects of alcohol use on the body are well understood. Excessive use increases risk for disease in the central nervous, cardiovascular, gastrointestinal, and immune systems and causes several types of cancers and nutrient deficiencies. Addiction to alcohol is a leading cause of malnutrition in developed countries (Lieber 1984, 2003). Primary and secondary malnutrition as a result of alcohol addiction are summarized in Table 20–3.

TABLE 20–3. Malnutrition resulting from alcohol addiction

Primary malnutrition

Empty calories are consumed (alcohol replaces usual nutrients).

Socioeconomic effect of addiction reduces nutritional intake.

Appetite is impaired.

Secondary malnutrition

Absorption is decreased in small intestine.

Use of nutrients by liver is impaired.

Degradation of nutrients in liver is increased.

Energy wasting occurs.

Primary malnutrition in the alcoholic patient is caused by a poor diet influenced by the socioeconomic effect of addiction and the tendency of alcohol to affect dietary carbohydrate intake. When caloric intake of alcohol exceeds 30% of a 2,000-kcal diet, carbohydrate, protein, and fat intake decrease significantly and may be associated with decreased intake of vitamins A, C, and B_1 (thiamine) and minerals (Lieber 2003).

Secondary malnutrition is caused by alcohol's direct effect on the liver and small intestine. Deficiencies in vitamins B_1, B_2 (riboflavin), B_6 (pyridoxine), C (ascorbic acid), D, K, E, and B_9 (folic acid) correspond to the amount of alcohol consumed. Vitamins A, E, and D are typically absorbed via dietary fats and are affected by impaired fat absorption secondary to alcohol consumption. Mineral deficiencies also result secondarily from the toxic effects of alcohol on the human body and include calcium, zinc, magnesium, iron, and selenium deficiencies (National Institute on Alcohol Abuse and Alcoholism 1993). Vitamin A deficiency is well understood in the cirrhotic patient.

Dietary recommendations in the alcoholic patient with nutritional deficiencies aim to

- Reduce the toxic effects of alcohol on the body
- Reduce inflammation with anti-inflammatory foods and supplements
- Improve the quality of foods ingested

The following nutritional recommendations are specific to the alcoholic patient:

- Encourage moderation or abstinence from alcohol.
- Encourage a balanced diet.
- B_1 (thiamine) 50–100 mg/day in active drinkers (prevents Wernicke-Korsakoff syndrome)
- B_2, B_6, minerals (via multivitamin); consider vitamin B-100/vitamin B-complex with extra thiamine.
- Dietary folate: best source is leafy greens; consider methyl folate supplement (the bioactive form; 30%–40% of population are estimated to have an impairment in the enzyme needed to make active folate), or add vitamin B-complex with active folate.
- Emerging antioxidant-focused therapies:
    - N-Acetylcysteine: may help restore glutathione levels; theoretically beneficial; evidence is limited.

- SAMe (*S*-adenosylmethionine): thought to oppose free radical production, shown to attenuate alcoholic liver injury in animal studies (Purohit et al. 2007); evidence is insufficient to support prevention or attenuation of liver disease in humans.
- Silymarin (milk thistle 160 mg one to three times per day): traditionally used for liver disorders; this herb may regenerate liver cells, protect the liver from toxic injury, improve liver function, and reduce risk of death from liver disease; evidence is mixed.

Nutrition and Other Substance Use

Beyond opioids and alcohol, data are limited for nutritional needs of patients with other substance use disorders. In general, we would suggest the anti-inflammatory diet with sufficient protein for all patients in recovery from substance use disorders as a reasonable health-promoting diet.

SUMMARY OF NUTRITION RECOMMENDATIONS

Tailor nutritional counseling to stages of use and recovery:

- *Active use or reduced use:* Encourage basic multivitamin for baseline nutritional delivery to address poor eating habits.
- *Early recovery (1–3 months) or moderate use:* Continue daily nutritional supplementation. Begin nonjudgmental inquiry about eating patterns and healthy choices patient is interested to make. Explore how cessation or moderation of substance use affects food choices, appetite, sleep, and weight.
- *Prolonged sobriety (6–12 months) or stable moderate use:* Deepen inquiry around patient's food choices, meal planning, and shopping and effects of food choices on quality of life.

Encourage all patients in recovery to move toward a whole foods–based anti-inflammatory diet with adequate protein.

Exercise

A sedentary lifestyle brings an increased risk for developing cancer, insulin resistance, heart disease, and mood disorders and has an effect on addiction and recovery. Alternatively, exercise benefits the patient regarding aspects of addiction and recovery.

Exercise can include aerobic activities (e.g., running and swimming), low-impact activities (e.g., hiking and walking), or mind-body activities (e.g., tai chi, yoga, and qi gong). The benefits of exercise are many:

- Improved mood and cardiac health
- Reduced stress and total cholesterol
- Increased endogenous "feel good" hormones, circulation, and oxygenation
- Toned muscles needed for stabilizing joints and balance

Clinical comment: For active substance users, suggest a simple activity like walking. Patients stable in their sobriety are better candidates for increased activity and may more easily experience its benefits: improved mood, decreased stress, improved sleep, decreased anxiety, and improved eating habits.

EVIDENCE IN SUBSTANCE USE DISORDERS

Exercise is known to have positive effects on stress levels, sleep, anxiety, and depression. It is also understood to act on the same reward pathways as drugs of abuse. Exercise produces the following effects:

- Increases dopamine receptor binding
- Decreases glutamate
- Enhances brain plasticity through chromatin (brain-derived neurotrophic factor) remodeling

This shared pathway with drugs of abuse highlights the "addictive" nature of exercise when practiced in excess and how chronic excessive exercise exposure (in animal studies) may resemble chronic exposure to drugs and lead to sensitization of the reward pathway.

PREVENTING DRUG INITIATION

Exercise appears to protect against the transition from initial use to addiction, as well as reduce drug intake in drug-dependent individuals. Various studies suggest the following (Lynch et al. 2013):

- Exercise may protect against adolescent drug use initiation, particularly cigarettes and illicit drugs.
- In animal studies, exercise decreases the reinforcing effects of substances such as alcohol, methamphetamine, cocaine, and opioids.
- A history of modest exercise appears to protect against later drug use. Chronic high-level exercise may enhance later vulnerability.

REDUCING CRAVING

Studies have shown that light-to-moderate exercise

- Helps reduce cravings for cigarettes.
- May help reduce cravings in patients with cannabis use disorder (Buchowski et al. 2011).

IMPROVING WITHDRAWAL SYMPTOMS

Currently, little is known about the effects of exercise on withdrawal from drugs of abuse in humans. However, animal research suggests that light to moderate exercise (Lynch et al. 2013)

- Improves nicotine withdrawal symptoms.
- Decreases stress, anxiety, and depression during withdrawal.
- Decreases hyperalgesia during morphine withdrawal.
- Protects against alcohol withdrawal seizures.

Qi gong has been shown to reduce opioid withdrawal symptoms (Li et al. 2002).

AIDING RELAPSE PREVENTION

Human studies on exercise as an adjunct to treatment show benefit in the following ways:

- Moderate intensity aerobic exercise as an adjunct to substance abuse treatment demonstrated an increase in percent days abstinent for both alcohol and drugs at the end of treatment (Brown et al. 2010).

- Exercise when combined with a smoking cessation program significantly increases abstinence rates (Ussher et al. 2014).

In several publications, Alan Marlatt explored the utility of exercise in improving outcomes in alcohol use and showed its benefit as a tool for relapse prevention (Murphy et al. 1986). Marlatt suggests that exercise can be incorporated as a means to (Larimer et al. 1999)

- Improve mood
- Develop self-efficacy
- Replace negative behaviors with positive ones, thereby rewarding and promoting a balanced life
- Encourage acquisition of skills, via yoga, hiking, and tai chi, with others in recovery

POSSIBLE LIMITATIONS OF EXERCISE

Animal and human models have shown that exercise (Lynch et al. 2013)

- May not be effective in reducing methamphetamine use after use has already begun
- May lead to higher levels of consumption (in one animal study examining the effect of exercise on binge drinking)
- May have gender- or substance-specific variations: running may be more effective in reducing initiation of use in females and decreasing preference for cocaine in males

SUMMARY OF EXERCISE RECOMMENDATIONS

Although the body of evidence is small, evidence supports exercise as a tool for preventing initiation, decreasing cravings and withdrawal symptoms, and aiding relapse prevention. Thirty minutes of moderate exercise three times per week is a reasonable adjunct to standard addiction treatment to support acute and long-term recovery.

KEY POINTS

Assess a patient's nutritional status, and consider the stage of recovery when making recommendations.

Integrate the anti-inflammatory diet with moderate protein.

Encourage mild to moderate exercise, noting that there may be different effects dependent on gender, type of substance, exercise history, and stage of recovery.

Use appropriate supplements for common nutrient deficiencies in specific substance use disorder patients.

References

Barnes PM, Powell-Griner E, McFann K, et al: Complementary and alternative medicine use among adults: United States, 2002. Adv Data 2(343):1–19, 2004 15188733

Brown RA, Abrantes AM, Read JP, et al: A pilot study of aerobic exercise as an adjunctive treatment for drug dependence. Ment Health Phys Act 3(1):27–34, 2010 20582151

Buchowski MS, Meade NN, Charboneau E, et al: Aerobic exercise training reduces cannabis craving and use in non-treatment seeking cannabis-dependent adults. PLoS One 6(3):e17465, 2011 21408154

Chen D, Liu Y, He W, et al: Neurotransmitter-precursor-supplement intervention for detoxified heroin addicts. J Huazhong Univ Sci Technolog Med Sci 32(3):422–427, 2012 22684569

Evangelou A, Kalfakakou V, Georgakas P, et al: Ascorbic acid (vitamin C) effects on withdrawal syndrome of heroin abusers. In Vivo 14(2):363–366, 2000

Larimer ME, Palmer RS, Marlatt GA: Relapse prevention: an overview of Marlatt's cognitive-behavioral model. Alcohol Res Health 23(2):151–160, 1999 10890810

Li M, Chen K, Mo Z: Use of qigong therapy in the detoxification of heroin addicts. Altern Ther Health Med 8(1):50–54, 56–59, 2002 11795622

Lieber CS: Alcohol-nutrition interaction: 1984 update. Alcohol 1(2):151–157, 1984

Lieber CS: Relationships between nutrition, alcohol use, and liver disease. Alcohol Res Health 27(3):220–231, 2003 15535450

Lynch WJ, Peterson AB, Sanchez V, et al: Exercise as a novel treatment for drug addiction: a neurobiological and stage-dependent hypothesis. Neurosci Biobehav Rev 37(8):1622–1644, 2013 23806439

Morabia A, Fabre J, Chee E, et al: Diet and opiate addiction: a quantitative assessment of the diet of non-institutionalized opiate addicts. Br J Addict 84(2):173–180, 1989 2720181

Murphy TJ, Pagano RR, Marlatt GA: Lifestyle modification with heavy alcohol drinkers: effects of aerobic exercise and meditation. Addict Behav 11(2):175–186, 1986 3526824

National Institute on Alcohol Abuse and Alcoholism: Alcohol and Nutrition. Alcohol Alert No. 22 PH 346 October 1993. Bethesda, MD, National Institute on Alcohol Abuse and Alcoholism, 1993

Nazrul Islam SK, Jahangir Hossain K, Ahmed A, et al: Nutritional status of drug addicts undergoing detoxification: prevalence of malnutrition and influence of illicit drugs and lifestyle. Br J Nutr 88(5):507–513, 2002 12425731

Purohit V, Abdelmalek MF, Barve S, et al: Role of S-adenosylmethionine, folate, and betaine in the treatment of alcoholic liver disease: summary of a symposium. Am J Clin Nutr 86(1):14–24, 2007 17616758

Ussher MH, Taylor AH, Faulkner GE: Exercise interventions for smoking cessation. Cochrane Database Syst Rev 8(8):CD002295, 2014 25170798

Index

*Page numbers printed in **boldface** type refer to boxes, figures, or tables.*

Anxiety, or anxiety disorders
alcohol and, 42, 44, **45, 47,** 50,
58, 59
anabolic-androgenic steroids
and, 74
benzodiazepines and, **87,** 88,
89, 91, 92–93
caffeine and, 100, 101, 105,
107
cannabis and, **111, 112, 113,**
118, 119, 123
cognitive-behavioral therapy
and, 262, 264
exercise and, 332
gambling and, 246, 250, 253
hallucinogens and, 129, 141,
142, 149
inhalants and, 161, 164
mindfulness and, 311, 313,
314, **331,** 331
opioids and, **181,** 185, 187,
194
stimulants and, **207,** 207,
210
tobacco and, **221, 227**
Anxiolytics, screening tests for
use of, 32. *See also*
Benzodiazepines
ASSIST (Alcohol, Smoking and
Substance Involvement
Screening Test), 14
Asthma, tobacco use and, 237
Athletes
coffee and, 107
use of anabolic-androgenic
steroids, 78
Attachment, 319
Attention-deficit/hyperactivity
disorder, drug screening
tests and, 33
Atypical hallucinogens, 130, 133,
135, 137, **138–139, 142, 150–
151.** *See also* "Designer
drugs," MDMA;
Salvinorin A
AUDIT (Alcohol Use Disorders
Identification Test), 53, **54**

Auditory disturbances, alcohol
withdrawal assessment
and, **45**
Automatic thoughts, 264–265,
265
AVE (abstinence violation
effect), 274–275, **275**

"Bagging," 158
BAL (blood alcohol level), 40
intoxication and, 42
Balance, in geriatric patients, 12
Bang, 155
Barbiturates, screening tests for
use of, 32
Barriers to care, 17–18
"Bath salts" (synthetic
cathinones), description of,
202
Bayer, 171
Beans, **128**
Beck, Aaron T., 259. *See also*
Cognitive-behavioral
therapy
Beers Criteria (2015), 81, 94
Behavioral addictions, 9–10,
243–244. *See also* Gambling
management, 254–255
Benzodiazepines, 10, 81–96
addiction
recognition of, 89–91
treatment, 92
for alcohol withdrawal, 47–48
comorbidities
medical, 93
psychiatric, 92–93
DSM-5 diagnostic criteria for
sedative, hypnotic, or anxiolytic intoxication, **85**
sedative, hypnotic, or anxiolytic use disorder,
90–91
sedative, hypnotic, or anxiolytic withdrawal, **87**
equivalency doses and half-
lives of, **48**
in geriatric patients, 89, 94